PLD The Liver
Polycystic Live

by Danevas

approx
54 g protein
doc says - approx 70 g

About PLD Liver Diet   8
Preparing Your Own Foods   11
What Is The PLD Diet?   12
Testing Alkalinity   17
Salt   21
Water   23
DNA   24
Enjoy These Items With PLD   28
Useful Grains Beans Nuts With PLD   63
Useful PLD Trials   72
Some Other PLD Useful Things   73
Better Protein Choices With PLD   74
Useful Drinks With PLD   82
Avoid These Items With PLD   144
Avoid Herbs With PLD   155
Avoid Chemicals With PLD   177
Everyone To Avoid   179
Avoid Drinks With PLD   180
Menus   188
Helpful Websites   197
Dermatology Symptoms   198
Alkaline Clinical Trial   201
PLD Pain   204
The Future   205

Copyright

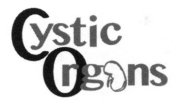

Fourth Edition

ISBN 9781521107270

Dedication

This is dedicated to the fine doctors who have studied PLD and have taken the time to research and understand PLD Polycystic Liver Disease. With this understanding, they have treated us, giving us many medical options.

This is also dedicated to individuals with PLD Polycystic Liver Disease who do not know where to turn, where to seek help, where to go once they receive the diagnosis of PLD.

Hormones, caffeine, chemicals (like bleach, herbicides. pesticides, xenoestrogens, endocrine disruptors) all can increase PLD symptoms. This book contains a detailed lists of items to be enjoyed and those to be avoided to maintain PLD Health.

Foreword

A single drop of water does not make a river.

~Author Unknown

I wish to thank those people whose contributions to this project have been invaluable with the artwork, with the text, with the proof-reading, with the layout and more. I also wish to acknowledge those participants who have sent me their feedback about their willingness to try this diet and lifestyle changes. It is all part of a vast experiment that we are embarking on together. We have opened the doorway toward health.

About PLD Liver Diet

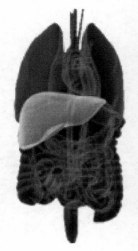

Inside the confines of your own personal health, what follows are guidelines to try to incorporate into your care, checking first with your own physician before implementing.

Plant based Diet Geared To Liver Health

Protein 0.6 grams/kg

1200 mg Sodium

4 liters Water or Twice Urine Output

Low Fat

Food Restriction

Polycystic Liver Disease PLD is an inherited disease that causes smooth liver tissue to fill with numerous fluid filled balloon like cysts. The fluid within these cysts is found to be the same fluid as in the plant coleus. This is also known as Forskolin.

Some have even gone on a raw food vegan diet This has shown great promise in reducing liver size. Try to eat some raw fruits and vegetables each day. Or try juicing these same vegetables or fruits. Wait 20 minutes following any citrus before attempting to eat something else.

These cysts multiply. In severe cases, liver cysts are the cause of massive liver enlargement This is called severe symptomatic hepatomegaly. Researchers measured several livers with MRI both from normal people without any liver disease and several patients with PLD Polycystic Liver Disease.

The result is that each person has the exact same amount of normal functioning non-cystic liver. Cystic liver is non functioning liver. This is why, in part, the liver continues to grow and expand. The liver is attempting to maintain a set amount of functioning liver. The liver is the only organ within the human body that is capable of this type of regeneration.

By the liver size growing and expanding, a cystic liver can reach a weight of greater than 40 pounds. The sheer size of a PLD liver compresses many of the internal organs. This can result in afflicted people seeking out some type of a debulking procedure, such as a liver resection, a TAE, or an organ transplant. We are very lucky in that a PLD liver seldom fails. Some with PLD have tried the experimental drug octreotide to decrease their liver size.

It is not a cure for Polycystic Liver Disease that we are seeking. We are collectively asking the answer to the following question,

"How can we maintain the health of a polycystic liver or our transplanted organs?"

Preparing Your Own Foods

Cooking all foods yourself, without using canned, bottled or prepared substances, is greatly influential in eating healthier. Couple this with carefully choosing locally grown, non-GMO (non genetically engineered) produce, that is in season; purchased at its peak ripeness, organic or preferably local, can also positively influence polycystic health.

If you have the ability or the inclination to grow your own fruits and vegetables, this too has many added benefits.

Some mass produced foods (i.e., vegetables, chicken, etc.) are dipped in a bleach bath before coming to market or picked green or grown especially to be transported instead of for taste or nutritional content.

Other animal proteins have questionable processes performed. Lear more about this through viewing these interesting food documentaries:

HELPFUL FOOD DOCUMENTARIES

Food, Inc.
Super Size Me
Food Revolution LA
The China Study
No Happy Cows
Forks Over Knives
Best Diet

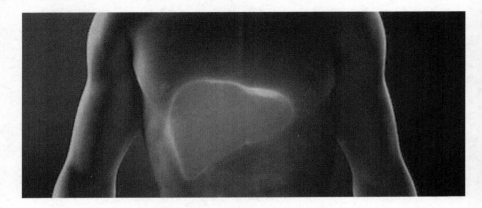

What Is The PLD Diet?

By incorporating dietary and lifestyle changes many have successfully diminished countless PLD Polycystic Liver Disease symptoms, including those of painful events and bloating episodes. Some have experienced an increase in energy and a lucky few have noticed an improvement in liver functioning as they age, though with polycystic liver disease, functioning rarely declines. And a further group of individuals have noticed that their PLD has decreased in size.

Some pages contain lists of items to be enjoyed and to be avoided. To find out the reasons try this website:

http://www.AlkalineDiet.com

HELPFUL WEBSITES

http://www.PKDiet.com/index2.php

TO HELP MAINTAIN PLD HEALTH:

Monitor alkalinity~maintain an alkaline urinary pH

Monitor BP Blood Pressure at or below 119/79

Enjoy eating a diet that maintains neutral protein

Monitor urinary protein

1200 mg sodium diet (salt)

Drink 4 liters of water/day

Decrease stress: find a room, a place where you can relax

Maintain movement each day, i.e. daily walks, Tai Chi

Avoid Liver Toxins: yeast, alcohol, ammonia

Avoid Xenoestrogens

Avoid Phytoestrogens

Avoid Bleach, Hormones

Avoid Sugars

PLD diet is a possibility for others to try to see if it might work as well as it has for some of us with PLD. Individual health issues are known by you. These pages are meant as guides, as suggestions for you to try. Alkaline foods generally are fruits and vegetables; enjoy these freely. Acidic foods are animal proteins, these are limited. There are some exceptions.

Generally the sweeter the taste of a raw fruit or vegetable, the more alkaline producing it is.

Besides animal proteins causing acidity, other acid producing culprits are concentrated sugars and alcohols.

Alcohol ferments are extremely harmful for PLD. These are ferments from wine, alcohol, yeasted baked goods.

A loaf of bread baked by you without any additional yeast will squelch symptoms.

Thus far, through self-testing, a usable alkaline sweetener seems to be tupelo honey or by adding dried fruits, bananas, dates, raisins, or cinnamon this can also lend sweetness to a dish. Recipe inspirations can be found at the website PKDrecipes.com.

When you prepare foods yourself, you know what is contained within it. You know what you have added or omitted to a dish.

Foods prepared with concentrated sugars bypass the hungry center of the brain and they have been known to cause urinary pH to register acidic (pH 5), raise serum cholesterol, create mood swings, increase cystic organ symptoms, and oftentimes trigger the onset of a painful headache even a migraine.

If one can eliminate animal proteins, and continue to obtain a daily intake of essential amino acids and essential fatty acids, this is better for polycystic organ health.

Essential fatty acids are those needed to replenish each day. Some vegetable food sources of essential fatty acids are chia, hempseed, and purslane.

Vegetables that contain sulfurins, typically contain many of the essential amino acids to be consumed daily: i.e., broccoli, Brussel sprouts, cabbage, turnips, or rutabagas. Juicing of these vegetables helps increase the amount of essential amino acids absorbed. Young cereal grasses also can contribute an amino acid rich juice. The molecule for heme from hemoglobin, looks very similar to the spelt grass juice molecule. Drinking cereal grass juices may help correct anemia. Foods can really make a difference in how one feels with PLD Polycystic Liver Disease. Buddha's hand is grown is a county of Japan. The villagers use Buddha's hand to replace all the starch in their diet including rice. The people of this county have better than the average health and they have never suffered from liver disease.

Other sources of proteins are grains, nuts, seeds, legumes, and beans, all soaked to diminish their phytic acid content. Spelt has the highest protein source of all the grains and lowest amount of phytic acid. Whereas wheat has been modified by commercial farming techniques and contains the highest amount of phytic acid of all the grains. Sprouts, especially sprouted grains are high in amino acids. If one is gluten intolerant, some useful grains are arrowroot, tapioca flour, bean flour, sunchoke flour or brown rice flour~caution rice has higher levels of arsenic.

Foods containing leucine are particularly good for us.

Another possibility is for one to limit the daily intake of animal proteins to three ounces or less; no more often than two or three times a week. The size of a deck of cards corresponds to about three ounces of fish. One dice is the equivalent of one ounce of cheese.

Ingesting animal proteins can also adversely affects PLD Polycystic Liver Disease.

This act increases stomach acids, changing the pH of digested chyme. This change stimulates the release of secretin, a known liver cyst growth trigger which is capable of expanding liver cysts from flat envelopes into round bubbly cysts.

Hormones can directly increase liver cyst size. With severe PLD Polycystic Liver Disease, alternatives to pregnancy are oftentimes discussed. Consider switching from coffee to a roasted grain beverage. Caffeine, even in minute amounts, increases all cyst growth.

The PLD Diet

- Plant based alkaline diet geared to Liver Health:
  Test urinary pH at night.

- Neutral Protein 0.6 grams/kilogram:
  Test your own to get an idea of how much protein is necessary.

- 1200 mg sodium, Low fat:
  Take your own blood pressure in the morning keep it below 119/79.

- 4 liters of water or twice urinary output:
  Shut down your own vasopressin

- Low fat:
  Eat a low fat diet.

- Food restricted:
  Food restrict whenever possible.

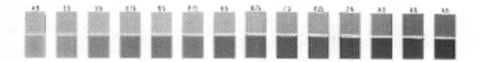

Testing Alkalinity

• Plant based alkaline diet geared to liver health
Test Urinary pH at night.

Using nitrazine paper, a dipstick, or pH paper on a roll (Vivid with a range of 5.5 - 8.0) self-testing of urinary pH is possible.

To test urinary pH: Do so at night, the last thing before going to sleep–Tear a piece of pH paper and pass the torn paper strip through your urine stream.

Read and compare the color change against the provided chart to determine your urinary pH. Another method is to urinate into a disposable cup and dip pH nitrazine paper into the urine.

If using pH paper on a roll is more to your liking, Micro essential labs stocks the most commonly requested #067 with a range of 5.5 to 8.0 - 3 roll refills. Amazon also carries this. Testing pH dipsticks are available from pHion and Micro essential and are thought to be easier to read.

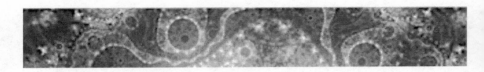

Neutral Protein

- Neutral Protein 0.6 grams/kilogram

Test your own urinary protein between doctor's visits.

<u>Calculate Neutral Protein</u> Multiply kilograms of body weight by 0.6 grams of protein.

1 kilo = 2.2 #s

110 pound person: multiply 50 kg by 0.6 = 30 grams of protein per day.

176 pound person: multiply 80 kg by 0.6 = 48 grams of protein per day.

Neutral protein is achieved when the amount of protein eaten daily is equal to the amount that comes out, called a neutral balance. Eating extra protein puts weight on plus it unnecessarily increases the burden of the workload on kidneys.

Neutral protein is 0.6 grams of protein per kilogram of body weight. Eating a neutral amount of protein helps kidneys remain healthier and allows kidneys to more readily eliminate any toxins and acids from the body. This in turn keeps a PLD cystic liver healthy.

Eating proteins changes the stomach pH toward acidic. When it reaches a certain acidity, this will release secretin. Secretin is what triggers PLD liver cysts to fill with fluid and expand.

A protein <u>chart</u> has been prepared by a fellow PLD'r.
http://www.polycystic-kidneydisease.com/pdf/protein.pdf
This contains some protein values for certain foods. Do continue to limit animal protein to three ounces or less per day and no more often than two or three times a week.

Ingesting animal proteins adversely affects PLD Polycystic Liver Disease. This act increases stomach acids, changing the pH of digested chyme. This change stimulates the release of secretin, a known liver cyst growth trigger which is capable of expanding liver cysts from flat envelopes into round bubbly cysts.

Hormones can directly increase liver cyst size. With severe With PLD Polycystic Liver Disease, alternatives to pregnancy are oftentimes discussed.

Consider alternatives to pregnancy. Consider switching from caffeine beverages like tea or coffee to a roasted grain beverage. Caffeine, even in minute amounts, increases all cyst growth by increasing cyclic AMP which in turn increases cyst growth.

The proteins excreted in the urine are a different type with cystic organ disease than with other types of kidney disease. Eating a neutral protein diet will greatly aide this spillage especially as one continues to age.

Using certain blood pressure medications such as ACE inhibitors can also decrease protein spillage in the urine. A study was attempted with children who had ARPKD to stop the protein spillage before it began by placing them on very very low dose blood pressure medication.

Fish though thought to be healthy, is not healthy for a PLD liver. Fish are a food that is highest in mercury, pesticides, herbicides. Fish is so high in these harmful toxins that in many fishing regions the citizens will not purchase these fish.

Salmon, particularly farmed fish, are a source of disease. A salmon farm can hold upwards of 2,000,000 salmon in a relatively small amount of space. These overcrowded conditions result in disease, which spreads rapidly among the stressed salmon. To counteract these pesticides a neurotoxin is used. Testing has confirmed that farmed salmon contains the greatest amount of toxins of all and this is by an incredibly large margin. However most of the toxins come from the feed itself.

Other than salmon, there are so many other plant based foods to help increase omega 3's which is beneficial to PLD. These vegetable sources are hemp seed, purslane, chia seeds.

Continue to avoid flaxseed. Though high in omega 3's, flaxseed is a super endocrine disruptor. It is linseed. Linseed oil has been used as paint thinner, putty, wood finish, linoleum. Flax has been grown as a non food source, for paper, for cloth originally. As a non food source more pesticides and herbicides can be sprayed on flax then if it was only grown as a food source. Flax can cause your PLD cysts to grow and it increases liver pains. Because of the combination of growing and spraying of chemicals, this has allowed flax to become a super endocrine disruptor.

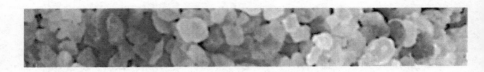

Salt

- Salt 1200 mg sodium

One-eighth teaspoon of salt is equivalent to 1200 mg of sodium. Due to the hidden salt in many prepared foods cooking your own food without salt, goes a long way to staying on a 1200 mg sodium diet.

Table salt contains aluminum to make it free flowing. Higher amounts of aluminum have been found in the brains of individuals with dementia and Alzheimer's. Try Himalayan pink crystal salt, limiting it to one-eighth teaspoon per day. If permitted, 2-5 drops of solé taken daily in a full glass of water seems to help some; read a few thoughts on solé.As we age systematically, by using Himalayan salt exclusively, we manage to maintain the exact same proportions of minerals from the chemical scale that are needed by the body.

Table salt contains aluminum. Aluminum is found in higher concentrations in the brains of autopsied corpses with Alzheimer's. Hawaiian researchers have discovered that those populations eating more soy tofu, more soy products go much more quickly toward dementia. This is thought to be due to aluminum pipes used in the commercial preparation of soy products. In other cases it has been due to the genetically modified soy bean. Humans unknowingly consume these GMO soy vegetables and other GMO fruits and vegetables.

Hawaiian researchers have discovered this by studying differences between the Asian cultures: the Japanese, the Filipinos, the Samoans, the Hawaiians, the Chinese, the Koreans, and others as it relates to health.

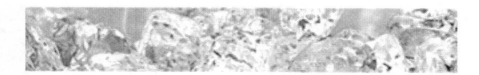

Water

- 4 liters of water or twice urinary output

If permitted, drink enough water to suppress vasopressin release. Vasopressin triggers cyst growth. Decreased cyst growth slows down PLD development and symptoms. Some are trying to drink twice their urinary output or approximately 4 liters of water per day. Others with liver cysts alone are using increased water intake to help flush the liver and keep it optimally functional.

A Low-Osmolar Diet clinical trial was undertaken at Tufts University in the USA. Four liters was the required amount of water to shut down vasopressin, a protein involved in cyst growth.

https://www.ncbi.nlm.nih.gov/pubmed/27663039

Researchers have concluded that drinking 4 liters of water in addition to other liquids (herbal tea, juice, etc.), will shut down vasopressin, a protein the signals cyst growth. A liter of water is approximately equal to a quart.

Only 8% of those with PLD Polycystic Liver Disease will require some help with their enlarging liver. Others will not be bothered by it at all.

DNA

Use all means possible to protect the integrity of your own DNA.

This squelches the probability of the second hit inheritance.

We each have inherited the gene for PLD Polycystic Liver Disease or PKD Polycystic Kidney Disease, but how it manifests in each of us is different, including how others within families may manifest PLD.

A few things that are best avoided with PLD:

- Ammonia / Window cleaner
- Alcohol: perfumes, windex, wine, beer, spirits
- Arginine
- Aspirin, Tylenol, NSAIDs, Advil, Ibuprofen can decrease liver function
- Animal products limit to no more than 3 ounces/day: 2-3 times/week
- Bleach: Clorox, bleached cleansers, chicken dipped in bleach
- Carrots and pre-cut vegetables dipped in bleach
- Chemicals: DDT, pesticides, herbicides, soap powder
- Caffeine: chocolate, coffee, tea, cola, soda, pop
- Chlorine, chloride, carbon tetrachloride, plastic BPA

- Dairy
- Flaxseed
- Fish oil, cod liver oil
- Herbicides
- Hormones: birth control pills, HRT, testosterone, estrogen, progesterone
- Liver toxic herbs, estrogenic herbs
- Nightshade plants
- Pesticides
- Phytoestrogens
- Soy
- Sugar
- Tea: black, green, white, de-caffeinated tea/ coffee, and certain herb teas
- Xenoestrogens

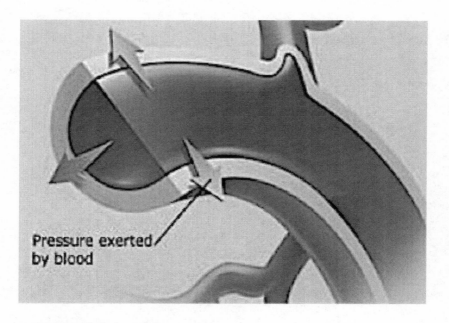

Pressure exerted
by blood

Blood Pressure

Test Blood Pressure in the morning.

Check your PLD blood pressure daily~in the morning when it is highest. Be sure it stays between 119/79. If it is out of this range, contact your physician and get help in maintaining a low blood pressure.

Other things to do are to:

Avoid allergic foods: soy, dairy, wheat.

Take daily walks.

Avoid caffeine.

For a more complete discussion try this website:

http://www.pkdiet.com/pkdBP.php

To follow are a list of foods to enjoy. Try this website to find out why.

http://www.AlkalineDiet.com/enjoy.html

Enjoy with PLD

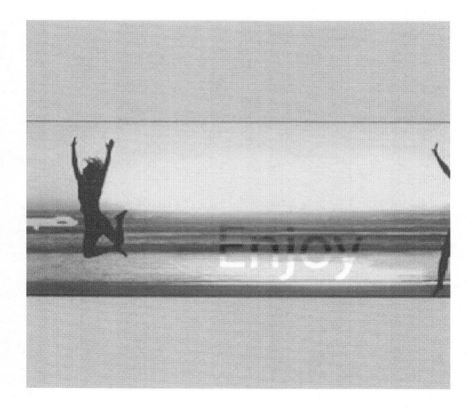

ENJOY WITH PLD

ACE

ACEi angiotensin converting enzyme inhibitors

Acerola

Acorn squash

Adzuki beans

Afinitor ® (everolimus)

Agaricus bisporus

Aging NMN

Albumin

Alkalinity

All fruit spread

Allium sativum

Almond butter

Almond milk (Ø carrageenan, sugar)

Almond milk ice cream ((Ø carrageenan, sugar)

Almond oil

Almond yogurt (Ø carrageenan, sugar)

Almond yogurt smoothie (Ø carrageenan, sugar)

Almonds

Amaranth

Amino acids (certain ones) can ↑ kidney functioning

Anasazi beans

Anti-inflammatory foods

ENJOY WITH PLD

Antibiotics if needed

Anutra

Aojiru

Apollinaris water

Apple

Apple banana

Apple cider Ø sugar

Apple concentrate as sweetener

Apple juice fresh

Apple sauce

Apples sweet

Apricot

Apricot juice

ARB angiotensin receptor site blockers

Arginex

Aronia

Aronia juice

Aronia melanocarpa

Arrowroot

Artichoke

Artichoke flour

Artichoke leaf

Artichokes globe

ENJOY WITH PLD

Artichokes Jerusalem

Artichokes sunchokes

Artocarpus altilis (breadfruit)

Arugula

Asparagus

Asteraceae

Autumn crocus only if needed by prescription

Avocado

Avocado oil

Baby spring greens

Badoit water

Bamboo shoots

Banana

Baps spelt

Barley

Barley grass

Barley grass juice

Barley milk (Ø carrageenan, sugar)

Barley powder

Bartlett pear

Bay leaf

Bean flour

Bean sprout noodles

ENJOY WITH PLD

Bean sprouts

Bean threads vermicelli

Beans all, soaked

Beans green beans

Beans soaked

Beans string, snap

Beef consommé

Beef restoran

Beef tea distilled

Beet juice

Beet tops ↑ oxalates

Beetroot

Bellis perennis

Bentonite clay

Berberine (wait)

Berries

Berry juice

Besan flour

Bilberry juice

Bing cherries

Bing cherry juice

Biodynamic

Bio magnet pairs

ENJOY WITH PLD

Biotin

Bitter melon

Black bean

Black currants

Black eyed peas

Black lentils

Black raspberry

Black rice

Black turtle beans

Blackberry

Blueberry juice

Blue Zones

Blueberry juice

Bok choy

Bon ami

Borax, laundry booster (do not inhale)

Boron

Borsec water

Boysenberry

Brassica

Brazil nuts caution arsenic

Bread Ø wheat yeast

Breadfruit

ENJOY WITH PLD

Breadnut

Breast milk

Brisdelle (paroxetine)

Broad beans

Broccoli

Broccoli DIMs

Broccoli rabe

Broccoli sprouts

Brown lentils

Brown rice caution arsenic

Brown rice noodles caution arsenic

Brussels sprouts

Bubble water

Buckwheat

Buckwheat noodles

Buckwheat sprouts

Buddha's hand

Burdock oil

Burdock root

Butter beans

Button mushroom

Cabbage

Cabbage Chinese

ENJOY WITH PLD

Cabbage juice

Cabbage red

Cabbage savoy

Calamansi

Caf-lib

Cafix

Calcium citrate

Calcium in vegan foods

Cannabidiol

Cannellini beans

Cantaloupe (local)

Cantharellus cibarius (chanterelle)

Caraway seeds

Cardoon

Caro

Carob

Carrot juice fresh

Carrots

Carum carvi (caraway)

Casaba melon

Cashews

Cassava, manioc, yuca root, tapioca

Cauliflower

ENJOY WITH PLD

CBD (cannabidiol)

Celeriac

Cellophane noodles

Cèpes mushrooms

Cereal grass juice

Chamomile

Chamomile tea

Chana flour

Chanterelle mushrooms

Chard

Charlotte's web

Chateldun water

Chayote squash

Cherimoya

Cherry

Cherry juice

Cherry Montmorency

Cherry sour

Cherry sour juice

Chestnut

Chia

Chia drink

Chia oil

ENJOY WITH PLD

Chia oil capsules

Chia seeds

Chickpea

Chickpea flour

Chico

Chicory

Chinese cabbage

Chinese peas

Chives

Chokeberry juice

Cilantro

Cinnamon

Citrus

Citrus juice fresh

Clear noodles

Clementine

Clementine juice fresh

Club soda

Coconut aminos

Coconut butter

Coconut especially young coconut spoon meat

Coconut flour

Coconut milk (Ø carrageenan, sugar)

ENJOY WITH PLD

Coconut milk ice cream (Ø carrageenan, sugar)

Coconut water

Coenzyme Q10

Coffee alternatives~roasted grains

Colchicine only if needed by prescription

Colchicum only if needed by prescription

Colgate wisp miniToothbrush

Collard greens

Colocasia esculenta (taro)

CoQ10

Corn bread organic Ø wheat sugar GMO

Corn meal organic

Corn organic Ø GMO

Corn salad nüssli mache

Corn tortillas organic Ø GMO

Cranberry Juice avoid the whole fruit

Creasy greens

Crêpes buckwheat Ø wheat

Crimini

Crookneck squash

Cruciferous vegetables

Cucumber juice

Cucumber Ø peel

ENJOY WITH PLD

Cumin

Curcumin

Currants

Curry leaf

Custard apple

Daikon radish

Daisy

Daiya

Dal

Dasheen araimo (taro)

Date sugar

Dates

Deadnettle

Delicata squash

DIMs (broccoli sprouts)

Dinkel

Donut peaches

Dr. Collins Restore toothpaste

Dragon fruit

Dried fruit

Drumstick plant

Dryland cress

Durian

ENJOY WITH PLD

Ecoplasts

Eddoes root

Edible flowers

Einkorn (spelt)

Elderberry juice

Elderberry syrup

Emmer (farro)

Emu oil

Endive chicory

English peas

Erythropoietin

Escarole

Farro

Fava beans

Ferrarelle water

Figs dried or fresh

Flageolets

Floradix

Fluoride carrageenan free toothpaste

Forbidden rice

Fresca Chia

Fruit

Fruit concentrate

ENJOY WITH PLD

Fruit dried

Fuji apples

Fuzzy toothbrush

GABA rice~caution ↑ arsenic

Gabi taro

Gac

Gala apples

Galangal

Ganoderma lucidum (Lingzhi/Reishi mushroom)

Garbanzo beans chick peas

Garbanzo flour

Garlic

Garlic oil

Gelatin

Gerolsteiner water

Ghassoul clay

Girasole

Globe artichoke

Gobi

Golden delicious apple

Golden raspberry

Gooseberry

Grain beverage barley brew

ENJOY WITH PLD

Grain beverage barley cup

Grain beverage cafix

Grain beverage caro

Grain beverage carob powder

Grain beverage inka

Grain beverage java herb uncoffee

Grain beverage kara kara

Grain beverage organic instant grain

Grain beverage Oshawa coffee

Grain beverage pero

Grain beverage prewetts chicory

Grain beverage roma

Grain beverage spelt kaffe

Grain beverage teeccino

Grain beverage yorzo

Gram flour

Grape

Grape concentrate

Grape juice

Grape seed

Grape seed extract

Grapefruit caution

Grapefruit juice caution

ENJOY WITH PLD

Gravenstein apples

Great northern bean

Green beans

Green brown lentils

Green juice

Greens collard

Greens kale

Greens leafy

Greens mustard

Greens purslane

Grits organic ø GMO caution aflatoxin

Groats

Guava

Gumbo file powder

H2 blockers (if needed)

Haricots verts

Harmless Hrvt coconut water

Hazelnut

Hazelnut milk

Hearts of palm

Helianthus tuberosus

Hemp seed

Hemp seed butter

ENJOY WITH PLD

Hemp seed milk (Ø carrageenan, sugar)

Hemp seed oil

Hemp seed oil capsules

Herb Tea bamboo

Herb Tea blood orange

Herb Tea burdock root

Herb Tea chamomile

Herb Tea chamomile citrus

Herb Tea hibiscus

Herb Tea lemon balm

Herb Tea lemon thyme

Herb Tea lemon water

Herb Tea lemongrass

Herb Tea lime leaf

Herb Tea linden flower

Herb Tea milk thistle

Herb Tea mint magic

Herb Tea nettle leaf

Herb Tea peppermint

Herb Tea rose hips

Herb Tea saffron

Herb Tea silymarin

Herb Tea soba

ENJOY WITH PLD

Herb Tea speedwell

Herb Tea sugar cookie sleigh

Herb Tea thyme

Herb Tea tilleul

Herb Tea veronica

Herb Tea watermelon seed

Hibiscus

Himalayan salt

Honeydew juice

Honeydew melon

Huckleberry juice

Injera

Inositol

Iron foods ↑ iron

Iron innate iron response when prescribed

Iskiate

Jack N' Jill toothpaste

Jackfruit

Jerusalem artichokes

Jicama

Kabocha squash

Kale

Kale Juice

ENJOY WITH PLD

Kamut

Kidney beans

Kiwi

Klettenwurzel haar oil

Kohlrabi

Komatsuna

Krachai

Kumquat

Lamb's lettuce

Lamium purpureum

Land cress

Langka

Lanreotide

Leafy greens

Leeks

Lemon

Lemon balm

Lemon egg

Lemon hot

Lemon juice freshly squeezed

Lemon thyme

Lemonade Ø sugar

Lemongrass

ENJOY WITH PLD

Lemons Meyer

Lentils

Lettuce butter

Lettuce curly leaf

Lettuce mache lamb's lettuce

Lettuce oak leaf

Lettuce romaine

Leucine

Lilikoi

Lima beans, butter beans

Lime

Lime flower tea

Lime juice

Lime leaf

Linden flower

Linden flower tea

Lingzhi

Liver useful

Long bean threads

Loquat

Lotus root

Lungkow vermicelli

Lutein

ENJOY WITH PLD

Lycopene

Mache lettuce

Magnesium (if OK)

Magnesium citrate (if OK)

Magnesium oil (if OK)

Magnet pairs

Malungai

Malunggay leaves

Mandarins

Mango

Mangosteen

Manihot esculenta, cassava

Manilkara zapota sapodilla (chico)

Manioc, cassava, yuca

Manuka bush

Manuka honey

Marjoram

Marrow beans

Marshmallow

Masa maize organic

Melissa cream

Melissa Extract Non-Alcoholic

Melon juice

ENJOY WITH PLD

Melon smooth skinned (local)

Menoquinone Ø Soy

Meso-zeaxanthin

Meyer lemons

Milk thistle silymarin

Millet

Millet soaked sprouted

Mineral water

Mint ↑ GERD

Miracle berry

Miraculin

Mixed wild greens

Mizuna

Mochi brown rice~caution ↑ arsenic

Montmorency cherry

Morchella

Morels

Moringa oleifera

Moroccan Red Clay

Mother's milk

Mulberry juice

Mung bean noodles

Mung bean sprouts

ENJOY WITH PLD

Mung beans

Murungai

Murungai leaves

Mushrooms edible

Mustard greens

Mustard seed

Myrtle

Naltrexone

Napa

Naringenin

Nasturtiums

Natto Ø Soy

Nattokinase Ø Soy

Naval oranges

Navy beans

Nectarines

Nettle ↓ uric acid

Nettle extract non alcoholic

Nettle leaf

Nexium

Niacin

Nicotinamide

NMN Nicotinamide Mononucleaotide

ENJOY WITH PLD

Northern beans

Nüssli (mache)

O3 Pure Ozone laundry

Oakleaf lettuce

Oat milk (Ø carrageenan, sugar)

Oats

Octreotide

Okinawan sweet potato

Okra

Olive caution ↑ salt

Olive leaf

Olive oil

Onion

Opo

Orange

Orange juice freshly squeezed

Orange lentils

Oregano ↓ candidiasis

Oyster plant

Pak choi

Papaya

Papaya juice fresh pressed

Paroxetine

ENJOY WITH PLD

Parsnip

Pasireotide (wait)

Passion fruit

Pasta (spelt kamut artichoke)

Pasta whole grain Ø wheat

Paw paw

Pea

Peach

Peach smoothies Ø sugar dairy

Pear

Pecans

Pellegrino water

Peppermint ↑ GERD

Pero

Perrier

Persimmon

Pineapple

Pineapple juice

Pink apples

Pinto bean

Pitihaya

Plantain

Polenta organic caution aflatoxin

ENJOY WITH PLD

Pomelo

Popcorn Ø salt organic caution aflatoxin

Porcini mushrooms

Portobello mushrooms

Potassium Citrate

Potatoes sweet

Potatoes sweet jewel

Potatoes sweet Okinawan

Prebiotics

Prilosec

Proteinuria ↓

Proton pump inhibitors

Pumpkin

Pumpkin seed oil

Purple archangel (red deadnettle)

Purslane

Queen Anne cherries

Quince

Quinoa soaked

Radish

Radish sprout

Rainier cherries

Raisin, organic

ENJOY WITH PLD

Ramon seed

Ramps

Rapamycin

Rapini

Raspberry caution pregnancy

Raspberry leaf

Raw local produce

Raw unheated coconut water

Red banana

Red bean

Red cabbage

Red cabbage juice

Red currants

Red deadnettle

Red kuri pumpkin

Red lentils

Red onion

Red rice (not yeast) caution arsenic

Reishi

Restore toothpaste

Rhassoul clay

Rhizomes

Rice crackers Ø wheat flax sugar yeast arsenic

ENJOY WITH PLD

Rice ice cream Ø carrageenan, sugar arsenic

Rice milk Ø carrageenan, sugar arsenic

Roasted grain tea

Romaine lettuce

Rose hips

Rutabaga

Rye

Rye bread Ø wheat yeast

Rye crackers Ø wheat yeast

Rye crisps Ø wheat yeast

Saffron ↓BP

Saffron tea

Sago root, sago tapioca pearls

Salsify, oyster plant, goatsbeard

Salt Himalayan limit

Sambucol

Samsca (caution liver)

San Pellegrino water

Sandostatin LAR

Sapodilla (chico)

Sapote

Saturn peach

Savoy cabbage

ENJOY WITH PLD

Scallions

Shallots

Shampoo Ø formaldehyde

Shampoo Ø methylisothiazolinone MIT

Shampoo Ø methyparabens

Shampoo Ø parabens

Shampoo Ø phthalates

Shampoo Ø sodium lauryl sulfate

Shea butter

Shohl's solution

Silymarin

Sirolimus

Slippery elm

Smooth skinned melons

Snap peas

Snow peas

Soba noodles Ø wheat

Soda water

Sodium Citrate

Solé

Sour cherry

Sour cherry juice

Speedwell

ENJOY WITH PLD

Spelt

Spelt bread

Spelt crackers Ø wheat flaxseed yeast

Spelt grass juice

Spelt pasta

Spelt stuffing Ø wheat

Spring water

Sprouts broccoli

Sprouts chickpea

Sprouts corn Ø GMO

Sprouts mung bean

Sprouts pea

Sprouts radish

Squash

Stem cells wait

Stinging nettle

String beans

Stuffing Ø wheat

Succotash

Summer savory

Sunchoke/flour

Swede

Sweet potato

ENJOY WITH PLD

Swiss chard

Tangelo

Tangerine

Tangerine juice

Tania root

Tapioca

Taro root gabi

Taste Nirvana coconut water

Teff

Test alkalinity

Test blood pressure

Test proteinuria

Thai ginger

Thyme

Thyme tea

Tight blood pressure control

Tilleul herb

Tilleul tea

Tolvaptan caution liver

Truffle

Tsamma juice

Tupelo

Tupelo honey

ENJOY WITH PLD

Turban squash

Turmeric

Turnip

Turnip greens

Ube

Ugli

Urtica dioica

Vanilla bean

Vanilla powder

Vasopressin suppression

Veg juice fresh

Vegan cream cheese

Vegetable korma

Vegetable pakoras

Velikdenche

Venlafaxine (Effexor)

Vermicelli clear

Veronica

Veronica tea

Vitamin B

Vitamin B complex

Vitamin B12

Vitamin B2

ENJOY WITH PLD

Vitamin B3 caution

Vitamin B6 (if prescribed caution)

Vitamin B7

Vitamin C

Vitamin D (if prescribed)

Vitamin E

Vitamin E oil

Vitamin K2 Ø Soy if prescribed

Walnuts

Washing soda

Water

Water chestnuts

Watercress

Watermelon

Watermelon juice

Watermelon seed tea

Wattwiller water

Wax beans

Welch onion, scallions

Wheat grass juice

White asparagus

White beans

White carrots

ENJOY WITH PLD

White mushrooms

White nectarines

White peaches

White radish

White yam

Whole grains organic Ø wheat

Wild onion ramps

Wild rice

Winter squash

Yams

Yellow currants

Yellow onion

Yellow squash

Yoga

Yuca

Zapota (chico)

Zeaxanthin

Zico coconut water

Zucchini Ø GMO

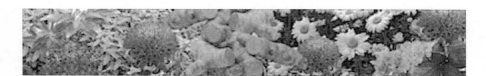

USEFUL HERBS WITH PLD

Acerola

Allium sativum

Aronia melanocarpa

Artichoke leaf

Asteraceae

Autumn crocus only if needed by prescription

Bay leaf

Bellis perennis

Bentonite clay

Bergamot

Berry

Bilberry

USEFUL HERBS WITH PLD

Brassica (mustard)

Breadnut

Cannabidiol

Caraway

Carob

Carcum carvi

CBD (cannabidiol)

Chamomile

Cherry

Chives

Chokeberry juice

Cilantro

Cinnamon ↑ GERD, helps regulate blood sugar

USEFUL HERBS WITH PLD

Colchicum only if needed by prescription

Cumin

Curry leaf

Daisy

Deadnettle

DIMs broccoli sprouts 👍

Elderberry

Galangal

Ganoderma lucidum

Garlic

Grapeseed

Gumbo file

Hempseed

USEFUL HERBS WITH PLD

Hibiscus
Himalayan pink salt
Krachai
Lamium purpureum (purple dead nettle)
Lemon balm
Lemon thyme
Lemon water
Lemongrass
Linden flower
Mallunggay leaves ↑ iron stores
Manuka honey
Marjoram
Marshmallow

USEFUL HERBS WITH PLD

Melissa
Milk thistle silymarin
Mint ↑ GERD
Moringa oleifera
Mustard seed
Myrtle
Nettle ↓ uric acid
Olive leaf
Oregano ↓ candidiasis
Peppermint ↑ GERD
Purple archangel (red deadnettle)
Purslane
Ramon seed

USEFUL HERBS WITH PLD

Raspberry leaf caution pregnancy
Rose hip
Saffron ↓BP
Saffron tea
Salt Himalayan limit
Sambuco
Shea butter
Silymarin
Slippery elm
Solé
Speedwell 👍
Stinging nettle
Summer savory

USEFUL HERBS WITH PLD

Tannia root
Thai ginger
Thyme
Tilleul
Tupelo
Turmeric
Urtica dioica
Vanilla bean
Vanilla powder
Velikdenche
Veronica
Watermelon seed

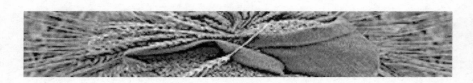

Enjoy Grains

USEFUL GRAINS BEANS NUTS
Adzuki bean
Almond butter
Almonds
Amaranth
Anasazi beans
Anutra
Arrowroot
Artichoke flour
Baps spelt
Barley
Bean flour

USEFUL GRAINS BEANS NUTS

Bean sprout noodles

Bean thread vermicelli

Beans soaked

Besan flour

Black bean

Black eyed peas

Black lentils

Black rice ~caution ↑ arsenic

Black turtle beans

Brazil nuts caution arsenic

Bread ∅ wheat yeast

Broad beans

Brown lentils

USEFUL GRAINS BEANS NUTS

Brown rice caution arsenic

Brown rice noodles caution arsenic

Buckwheat

Buckwheat noodles

Butter beans

Carob

Cashews

Cassava, tapioca, yuca root, manioc

Cellophane noodles

Channa flour

Chestnut

Chia

Chickpea

USEFUL GRAINS BEANS NUTS

Chickpea flour

Clear noodles

Coconut flour

Coffee alternatives

Colocasia esculenta (taro)

Corn bread organic Ø GMO

Corn meal organic Ø GMO

Corn starch noodles

Corn tortillas organic Ø GMO

Crêpes buckwheat Ø wheat

Dal

Dasheen araimo (taro)

Dinkel

USEFUL GRAINS BEANS NUTS

Einkorn (spelt)

Emmer (farro)

English peas

Farro soak

Fava soak and peel

Flageolets soak

Forbidden rice~caution ↑ arsenic

GABA rice~caution ↑ arsenic

Gabi taro

Garbanzo beans chickpeas

Garbanzo flour

Grain beverages

Gram flour

USEFUL GRAINS BEANS NUTS

Great northern bean

Green brown lentils

Grits organic Ø GMO

Groats

Hazelnut

Hempseed

Injera

Kamut

Kidney beans

Lentils

Lima bean

Long bean threads

Lungkow vermicelli

USEFUL GRAINS BEANS NUTS

Manihot esculenta, cassava

Marrow beans

Masa maiz

Millet

Mochi brown rice caution ↑ arsenic

Mung bean noodles

Mung beans

Navy beans

Northern beans

Oats

Orange lentils

Pasta spelt, kamut, rye Ø wheat

Pasta whole grain Ø wheat

USEFUL GRAINS BEANS NUTS

Peas
Pecans
Pinto bean
Polenta organic Ø GMO
Popcorn organic caution aflatoxin, Ø salt
Potatoes sweet
Potatoes sweet jewel
Potatoes sweet Okinawan
Pumpkin seeds
Quinoa
Red bean soak for 3 days
Red lentils
Red rice (not yeast) caution ↑ arsenic

USEFUL GRAINS BEANS NUTS

Rice crackers Ø wheat flax sugar yeast arsenic

Rye

Rye bread Ø yeast wheat

Rye crackers Ø yeast wheat

Rye crisps Ø yeast wheat

Sago root tapioca

Soba noodles

Spelt

Spelt bread Ø yeast

Spelt crackers Ø yeast flaxseed

Spelt pasta

Spelt stuffing Ø yeast wheat

Stuffing Ø wheat

USEFUL GRAINS BEANS NUTS

Sunchoke flour
Tapioca
Taro root
Teff
Vermicelli clear
Walnuts
White beans
White yam
Whole grains organic ø wheat
Wild rice
Yam
Yuca

ClinicalTrials.gov
A service of the U.S. National Institutes of Health

Useful PLD Trials

Possibly Useful, Still-in-Clinical-Trials-Medications https://goo.gl/ACzLfh
Afinitor® (everolimus)
Alkalinity
Bentonite clay
Octreotide - Somatostatin Sandostatin Lanreotide Pasireotide (wait for trial results)
Proton pump inhibitors
Potassium/sodium citrate
Rapamycin/sirolimus (wait for trial results completion)
Shohl's solution
Water

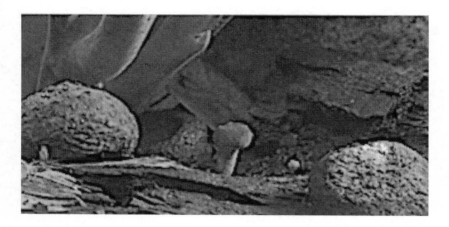

Some Other Useful Things For PLD

OTHER USEFUL THINGS
CLAY: Bentonite, pascalite, white, rhassoul, clay baths, soap, hair masques.
SAUNAS: Dry saunas, steam saunas, useful for sweating out body toxins.
MASSAGE: Gentle, relaxing massage.
REST: Restore yourself through rest: restorative yoga, gentle stretches, sleep.

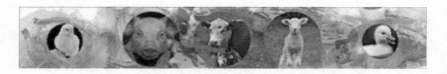

It is preferable to avoid animal proteins altogether. If you are unable to do this, limit animal proteins to 3 ounces/day, 2-3 times a week. If dairy or cheese is eaten, these are limited to one ounce, or approximately the size of one dice. Below are some better animal protein replacement suggestions. With cheeses and yogurts read labels carefully to assure they do not contain carrageenan.

Better Protein Choices With PLD

Better Protein Choices	Poorer Protein Choices
Daiya Vegan cheese	Blue cheese
Love my heart Vegan cheese	Blue veined cheeses
Almond cheese	Cottage cheese
Almond cheese	Ementhaler cheese
Daiya cheese	Feta cheese, salt-free, fat-free
Almond cheese	Goat cheese
Almond cheese	Paneer cheese
Almond cheese	Quark cheese
Coconut milk	Cow or goat milk

It is preferable to avoid animal proteins altogether. If you are unable to do this, limit animal proteins to 3 ounces/day, 2-3 times a week. If dairy or cheese is eaten, these are limited to one ounce, or approximately the size of one dice. Below are some better animal protein replacement suggestions. With cheeses and yogurts read labels carefully to assure they do not contain carrageenan.

Better Protein Choices	Poorer Protein Choices
Almond cheese	Sheep cheese
Coconut cheese	Soft white cheese
Almond milk lemon juice	Cultured buttermilk
Almond yogurt	Sour cream
Almond yogurt	Yogurt plain
Cultured Buttermilk	Whole milk
Cultured Plugra butter	Butter
Almond Yogurt plain cultured Ø carrageenan	Sour cream
Almond Yogurt Ø carrageenan + acidophilus	Yogurt with sugar or HFCS
Roquefort cheese	Parmesan
Swiss cheese	Romano cheese

Better Protein Choices	Poorer Protein Choices
Sheep cheese	Reggiani
Soft white cheese	Dry hard cheese
Blue cheese	Asiago cheese
Blue veined cheeses	Dry cheeses
Cottage cheese	Cheddar cheese
Dairy, cultured	Dairy, best avoided
Ementhaler	Orange yellow cheese
Feta salt free fat free	Mimolette cheese
Goat cheese	Mizithra cheese
Goat milk	Cow milk
Almond, rice, plant milk	Cow or goat animal milk
Paneer plant cheese	Cheddar cheese
Quark cheese	Kefalotyn

Better Protein Choices	Poorer Protein Choices
Lamb	Beef
Veggie burger Ø soy, Ø wheat	Hamburger
Halibut, Pacific	Salmon not farmed
Dover sole	Tuna
Perch	Sardines
Egg yolk: poached	Egg: fried, scrambled, white
Wild game	Commercial poultry
Wild turkey	Commercial turkey
Wild pheasant	Commercial pheasant

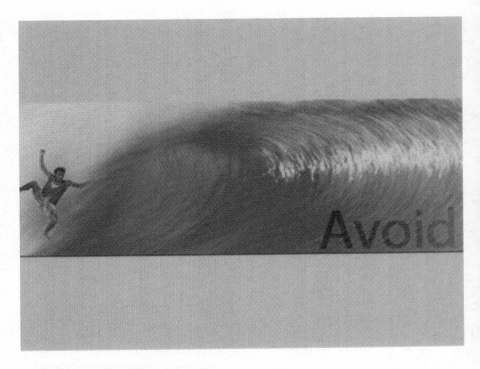

AVOID WITH PLD

To follow are items to be avoided. We know these increase PLD symptoms because each day we have measured our abdomen at the same point each morning and we have made note if these caused PLD pain.

ITEMS TO BE AVOIDED WITH PLD

3-benzylidene-camphor
4-Methylbenzylidene sunscn
Acacia fiber

ITEMS TO BE AVOIDED WITH PLD

Açai

Açai herb

Açai smoothie

Acesulfame potassium

Acetaminophen

Acetylsalicylic acid

Achyrocline

Ackee

Acrylamide

ADA azodicarbonamide

Advil

Aesculus hippocastanum

Aflatoxin

ITEMS TO BE AVOIDED WITH PLD

African autumn tea

African nectar tea

Agave

Agave cactus

Agave syrup

Aging (NMN)

Ahi tuna

Air fresheners phthalates

Alaskan king crab

Albacore tuna

Alcohol

Alcohol aerosols

Alcohol methanol

ITEMS TO BE AVOIDED WITH PLD

Aldomet

Ale

Aleve

Alfalfa sprouts

Algae

Alkylphenols

All purpose flour

Allspice

Almond ice cream (√ carrageenan)

Almonds with aflatoxin

Aloe vera (Ø eat)

Aluminum

Amalgam silver teeth fillings

ITEMS TO BE AVOIDED WITH PLD

Amino Acid L-arginine
Amino Acid L-canavanine
Amino Acid L-carnitine
Amiodarone
Ammonia
Anabolic steroids
Anchovies
Andouille sausage
Angelica dong quai
Animal proteins
Annatto
Anti-inflammatory medication
Antifreeze

ITEMS TO BE AVOIDED WITH PLD

Apple hard cider too much sugar, alcohol ferment

Apple pie/ Apple strudel

Arabitol

Arganat natural clay toothpaste

Arginine

Arsenic

Arstolochia

Artificial sweeteners

Ashwagandha

Asiago cheese

Aspartame

Aspergillus

Aspirin

ITEMS TO BE AVOIDED WITH PLD

Assugrin / Ashwagandha

Atrazine runoff in water supply

Atrazine weedkiller

Atta bulgur /durum / flour /

Aubergine

Auricularia polytricha (black fungus)

Autumn crocus only if needed by prescription

Aveeno nat mineral block face stick

Azodicarbonamide ADA

Bacon

Baguette wheat & yeast

Baked potato

Baking soda taken regularly

ITEMS TO BE AVOIDED WITH PLD

Bamboo rice~caution ↑ arsenic

Banana split

Basil

Bathroom sprays

BBQ

Bearberry

Beef

Beef / pork pies

Beef hot dog

Beer

Beet (if GMO)

Beet sugar (if GMO)

Bell peppers

ITEMS TO BE AVOIDED WITH PLD

BHA Butylated Hydroxyanisole

Bhatoora / Bhatura

BHT Butylated hydroxytoluene

Bihon

Bilberry whole fruit

Bio-oil

Birth control pills

Bisacodyl

Bisphenol A (BPA) plastic

Black cohosh

Black fungus

Black pepper caution aflatoxin

Black seed & oil

ITEMS TO BE AVOIDED WITH PLD

Black tea

Blackstrap molasses

Bleach

Bleach cleanser

Bleached flour

Blood dishes

Blue-green algae

Blueberry whole fruit

Bluefish ↑ mercury

Bologna

Bonito

Borage

Botanique toothpaste

ITEMS TO BE AVOIDED WITH PLD

Bottled juice methanol

Bovine growth hormone BGH

BPA

Bragg's liquid aminos

Brahmi

Brake fluid

Bratwurst

Brazil nuts caution aflatoxin

Bread flour

Bread pudding

Brinjal (eggplant)

Brown rice syrup caution ↑ arsenic

Brown sugar

ITEMS TO BE AVOIDED WITH PLD

Brownies

Buchu

Buckthorn

Bud-nip

Bulgur wheat

Bundt cake

Bust enhancing herbs

Butter

ButylatedHydroxyanisole BHA

Cacao

Cadmium

Caffeinated drink

Caffeine

ITEMS TO BE AVOIDED WITH PLD

Cake
Cake flour
Calendula
Callilepsis laureola
Calzone
cAMP
Canadian bacon
Canavanine
Candy
Cane juice
Cane juice crystals
Cane sugar
Canned goods ↑ methanol

ITEMS TO BE AVOIDED WITH PLD

Canned juice esp ↑ methanol

Canned meat/soups ↑ methanol BHT

Canned vegetables ↑ methanol

Cannelloni

Cannoli

Canola oil

Cantaloupe transported ridged melons develop fungus

Cape gooseberry (poha)

Capers

Cappuccino

Capsicum annuum

Carambola (starfruit)

Caramels

ITEMS TO BE AVOIDED WITH PLD

Carbamazepine

Carbon tetrachloride

Carbonated sodas

Carnitine

Carrageenan

Carrot cake

Carrots baby dipped in chlorine bath

Cascara sagrada

Casein

Cashew caution aflatoxin

Catchweed

Catfish

Cats claw

ITEMS TO BE AVOIDED WITH PLD

Catsfoot

Cayenne pepper

Celandine

Celery

Celery juice

Celery leaf

Cereal caution aflatoxin

Chaga mushroom/tea/powder

Chaparral

Chaparral tea

Chapati (wheat)

Charred meats

Chaste-tree berry

ITEMS TO BE AVOIDED WITH PLD

Cheddar cheese
Cheerios
Cheese
Cheese orange hard dry
Cheese parmesan
Cheese puffs
Cheeseburger
Cheesecake
Cheesesteaks
Chemicals ↑ cough
Chervil
Chicken dipped in chlorine bath
Chicken nuggets

ITEMS TO BE AVOIDED WITH PLD

Chicken sausage

Chili

Chinese gun powder tea

Chinese herbs

Chips salted

Chitosan

Chlorella

Chloride

Chlorine clorox comet

Chlorpropham

Chocolate

Chocolate cake/chip cookies / cookies / cupcakes/dipped strawberries / éclairs

Chocolate flourless cake / truffles /

ITEMS TO BE AVOIDED WITH PLD

Chocolate milk

Chokeberry whole fruit

Chondroitin

Chorizo

Chowder with dairy

Chrysanthemum tea

Cigarettes cigars chewing tobacco

Cimentidine

Clam & clam juice

Cleanser with bleach

ClearLax

Cleaver

Clenz-Lyte

ITEMS TO BE AVOIDED WITH PLD

Clotted cream
Cloud ear fungus
Clover / honey / sprouts
Cloves
Co-Lav
Coca cola
Cocktails
Cocoa
Coconut ice cream carrageenan/ Coconut oil/ Coconut sugar
Cod / Cod liver oil
Coffee/ Coffee beans ↑ estradiol 70%
Cohosh
Cola drinks / Cola nut

ITEMS TO BE AVOIDED WITH PLD

Colase®
Colax
Colchicine /Colchicum only if needed by prescription
Coleus
Colgate toothpaste
Colovage
Coltsfoot
Colyte
Comet cleanser
Comfrey
Commercial poultry dipped in bleach in USA
Concentrated sugar
Constipation

ITEMS TO BE AVOIDED WITH PLD

Cookies

Coral calcium

Coral white toothpaste

Cordarone (Amiodarone)

Cordyceps

Corn bread GMO caution aflatoxin

Corn dumplings GMO caution aflatoxin

Corn GMO caution aflatoxin

Corn syrup

Corned beef

Corydalis

Cosmetics phenoxyethanol

Cosmetics with cod liver oil

ITEMS TO BE AVOIDED WITH PLD

Cottonseed oil

Country mallow

Couscous

Crab

Cracker meal

Cranberry pills / whole fruit

Cream

Cream cheese

Cream of tartar

Cream puffs

Creatine supplements

Crème fraiche

Crest toothpaste

ITEMS TO BE AVOIDED WITH PLD

Crisco

Croissant

Crustaceans

Cupcakes

Custard

Cyclamate

Dairy

Dandelion greens

Danish

Daptacel vaccine (Phenoxyethanol)

Dark chocolate

DCA Dichloroacetate in tap water

DDD Dichlorodiphenyldichloroethane

ITEMS TO BE AVOIDED WITH PLD

DDE insecticide residue

DDT and residue

Decaf coffee

Decaf cola

Decaf drinks

Decaf tea

DEHP PVC plasticizer

Deli meat

Demerara sugar

Dessert concentrated sugars wheat

Detergents

Devil's claw

Dextrose

ITEMS TO BE AVOIDED WITH PLD

Dichloroacetate DCA

Dichlorodiphenyldichloroethane

Dieldrin insecticide

Diethyl phthalate

Diethylstilbestrol estrogen

Diflucan

Dill / Dill pickles

Diphenylthiazole DPT

Dong quai

Donuts

Doxidan

DPA

DPT

ITEMS TO BE AVOIDED WITH PLD

Dr. Pepper

Dreamsicle

Dried fruit caution aflatoxin

Dried plum

Dried prune

Dried strawberry

Dry cleaning clothing/chemicals

Dryer sheets

Dubliner cheese

Duck

Dulcolax

Durum

E-Z-Em Fortrans

ITEMS TO BE AVOIDED WITH PLD

Echinacea

Éclair

Ecstasy

Edamame

Eel

Egg /raw scrambled/ white

Eggnog

Eggplant

Elderberry whole fruit

Enchiladas

Endocrine disruptors

Endosulfane (insecticide)

Energy drinks

ITEMS TO BE AVOIDED WITH PLD

Enriched flour

Ensure

Ephedra sinica

Equal

Erythritol

Erythrosine FD C Red 3

Escargot

Espresso

Essiac

Estrace

Estrogen

Estrogen BCP/pill/patch

Estrogen disruptors / Estrogenic shampoo

ITEMS TO BE AVOIDED WITH PLD

Ethanol

Ethylene glycol

Eugenol (oil cloves)

Excedrin

Fabric softener

Face creams

Famotidine

Farina

Fennel

Fenugreek

Fermented products, fish paste

Fettuccine wheat

Figs dried caution alfatoxin

ITEMS TO BE AVOIDED WITH PLD

Filet mignon
Fish /anchovies /mackerel /sardines / trout/ tuna /salmon esp farmed / flounder
Fish oil /cod liver oil
Flagyl
Flax seed /crackers / oil capsules
Flour tortillas wheat
Fluconazole
Fluoride
Fo ti
Fontina cheese
Foods heated in plastic
Formaldehyde
Forskolin

ITEMS TO BE AVOIDED WITH PLD

Fragrance

Fragrance: BHT endocrine disruptor

Fragrance: Diethyl phthalate mimics hormones

Fragrance: Limonene can create formaldehyde

Fragrance: Octinoxate endocrine disruptor

Fragrance: Oxybenzone endocrine disruptor

Franks

French fries

Fried egg / egg white / foods / vegetables

Fructose

Fruit / Dried caution

Fudge

Fudgsicle

ITEMS TO BE AVOIDED WITH PLD

Galactitol

Ganoderma lucidum

Garcinia cambogia

GaviLax / GaviLyte

Gelatin

Gelato

Genistein (soy)

Gentamicin

Germander

Ghee

Ginger ↑BP / Ginger ale

Gingko biloba

Ginseng

ITEMS TO BE AVOIDED WITH PLD

Glechoma hederacea

Glucosamine

Glycols polyethylene (manufacture polyester)

GlycoPrep /Go-Evac / GoLytely

GMO genetically modified produce

Gnocchi

Goji berries nightshade

Golden seal root

Golden yukon potato

Goosegrass

Gotu kola

Graham crackers / flour

Grain beverage bambu

ITEMS TO BE AVOIDED WITH PLD

Grain beverage: postum (contains wheat)

Grain beverage: soy kaffee (contains soy)

Grain beverage: yannoh

Grape seed oil

Grapefruit / juice caution

Green leaf tea

Green rice caution ↑ arsenic

Ground meats, fish, poultry

Groundnuts aflatoxin

Groundsel

Grouper ↑ mercury

Guar bean / gum

Guarana

ITEMS TO BE AVOIDED WITH PLD

Hair dye chemicals / gel

HalfLytely

Ham / Ham hocks

Hamburger turkey burger, fish burger

Hard cheese

Harmful herb teas African Autumn

Harmful herb teas Bengal spice

Harmful herb teas black cherry berry

Harmful herb teas caffeine free

Harmful herb teas chaparral

Harmful herb teas cinnamon apple spice

Harmful herb teas country peach passion

Harmful herb teas cranberry apple zinger

ITEMS TO BE AVOIDED WITH PLD

Harmful herb teas fast lane black tea

Harmful herb teas honeyVanillaChamomile

Harmful herb teas lemon verbena ↓ herpes

Harmful herb teas lemon zinger

Harmful herb teas licorice root

Harmful herb teas mama bear's cold care

Harmful herb teas mandarin orange spice

Harmful herb teas morning thunder

Harmful herb teas raspberry zinger

Harmful herb teas red zinger

Harmful herb teas rooibos

Harmful herb teas rooibos chai

Harmful herb teas sleepytime kids grape

ITEMS TO BE AVOIDED WITH PLD

Harmful herb teas sleepytime peach

Harmful herb teas sleepytime vanilla

Harmful herb teas sweet apple chamomile

Harmful herb teas tangerine orange zinger

Harmful herb teas tension tamer

Harmful herb teas true blueberry

Harmful herb teas wild berry zinger

Harmful tea black

Harmful tea caffeine

Harmful tea Chinese gunpowder

Harmful tea decaffeinated

Harmful tea Earl Gray tea

Harmful tea green tea

ITEMS TO BE AVOIDED WITH PLD

Harmful white tea
Harpagophytum
Hash browns
Hawthorne ↑BP
Heating Food in microwave
Heptachlor (insecticide)
Herbicides
Herring
Hershey bars
HFCS High fructose corn syrup
Hoagies
Homocysteine
Hops

ITEMS TO BE AVOIDED WITH PLD

Hormones HRT

Horse chestnut

Horseradish

Horsetail

Hot chocolate

Hot dogs, rindswurst

Hot fudge sundae

Hot tamales with lard

Hot toddies

Huckleberry

Hydrogenated starch hydrolysate

Ibuprofen

Ice cream / drumstick

ITEMS TO BE AVOIDED WITH PLD

Iceberg lettuce
Imitrex
Impila root
Inflammation
Isomalt
Italian sausage
Jaggery
Jalapeño pepper
Jason Oral comfort toothpaste
Jason PowerSmile toothpaste
Jheri Redding texturizing gel
Jin Bu Huan
Juice bottled or canned (BPA)

ITEMS TO BE AVOIDED WITH PLD

Juniper berries

Just like sugar

Kava-kava

Keishi-bukuryo

Ketoconazole

Kiss my face toothpaste

Kola nut

Kombu (dashi, bonito flakes)

Kombucha

Krameria triandra (rhatany root)

Kudzu

Kwao krua kao

L-arginine

ITEMS TO BE AVOIDED WITH PLD

L-canavanine

L-carnitine

L'oreal HiP High Intensity Pigments

L'amour encage

Lactitol

Lady fingers

Langoustines

Lassi / Latté

Laundry powder

Lavender

Laxatives / Lax-a-Day / LaxLyte /

Lead

Lecithin (soy)

ITEMS TO BE AVOIDED WITH PLD

Lei gong teng (Wait)

Lemon verbena

Lesys (Maltitol, maltisweet, sweetPearl)

Licorice / drinks ↑ BP

Limonene→ formaldehyde

Lindane (insecticide)

Link sausage

Linseed / oil

Lithium

Liver & Liverwurst

Liver toxic herbs

Lobelia

Lobster

ITEMS TO BE AVOIDED WITH PLD

Loco moco
Lollipop
Longan
Luchi
Lupin
Lychee
Lysergic Acid LSD
LytePrep
Ma Huang
Maca
Macaroni salad /Macaroni and cheese
Mace
Macela achyrocline satureoides

ITEMS TO BE AVOIDED WITH PLD

Mackerel ↑ mercury

Macrogol

Magnolia Officinalis

Mai tai

Malasadas

Malt liquor

Maltitiol / Maltisweet (Maltitol Lesys SweetPearl) . Mannitol

Mangosteen juice

Manicotti

Maple syrup

Maraschino cherries

Margarine

Marlin ↑ mercury

ITEMS TO BE AVOIDED WITH PLD

Masala dosa w/wheat & potato

Maté

Matzo / Matza / Matzah

Meat red

Meatballs

Meatloaf

Mederma scar cream

Melaleuca

Melon transported ridged develop fungus

Menaquinone w/ soy

Mercury

Metalloestrogens

Methanol /Methanol alcoholic drinks

ITEMS TO BE AVOIDED WITH PLD

Methionine

Methoxychlor (insecticide)

Methyldopa

Methylisothiazoline DNA damage

Methylparabens

Mexican chocolate

Microwaved food / popcorn

Migraine

Milk / milk shakes /cow goat animal milks

Miraculin / Miracle berries

MiraLAX

Miso / Miso soup

Mistletoe

ITEMS TO BE AVOIDED WITH PLD

Mixed alcoholic drinks Methanol

MK-7 w/soy

Mochi white rice caution ↑ arsenic

Mochiko

Molasses

Monk fruit in the raw

Monster energy drink

Monterrey jack cheese

Motherwort

Motrin

Mountain apple

Movicol / MoviPrep

Mozzarella cheese

ITEMS TO BE AVOIDED WITH PLD

MSG monosodium glutamate

MSM (Methylsulfonylmethane)

Mulberry whole fruit

Mullet

Multiple vitamins

Muscovado

Mussels

Mycose

N-nitrosomorpholine NNM

Naan

Nail chemicals / Nail polish and removers

Naproxen

Nattō from soy / Nattokinase

ITEMS TO BE AVOIDED WITH PLD

Natural dentist toothpaste / Natural tea tree toothpaste

Neats foot oil

Nectresse

Neem toothpaste

Neotame

Neutrogena body oil / Neutrogena liquid facial cleanser fragrance free

Nigella sativa

Nightshade plants

Nitrites / Nitrosamine

Nizoral

Non-dairy creamer

Non-stick teflon

Noni juice & fruit

ITEMS TO BE AVOIDED WITH PLD

Nonylphenol derivatives

Norbu

NSAIDs

NuLYTELY

Nutmeg

NutraSweet

Nutribiotic toothpaste

Nutritional yeast

OCL (laxative)

Octinoxate sunscreen

Oil canola/coconut/cottonseed/grapeseed/lavender/safflower/sesame/sunflower

Oil, tea tree oil (melaleuca)

Oilseeds caution aflatoxin

ITEMS TO BE AVOIDED WITH PLD

Oily fish

Olay Daily Facials Deep Cleansing Cloths

Onion dip

Orange cheese

Orange roughy ↑ mercury

Organ meats

Organic chlorinated pesticides

Osha root

Ospemifene / Osphena

Oven cleaners

Oxybenzone

Packaged vegetables (chlorine bath)

PAHs Polycyclic aromatic hydrocarbons

ITEMS TO BE AVOIDED WITH PLD

Palm oil

Pancit

Panela

Papad / Pappadam

Paprika

Paraben

Paracetamol

Parmesan cheese / Parmigiano cheese

Parsley

Pasta wheat

Pastrami

Paté foie gras

Patis

ITEMS TO BE AVOIDED WITH PLD

Pau d'arco

Peanuts / butter / cookies /cups /pretzels aflatoxin

Pecans aflatoxin

Peg Lyte

Pemmican

Pennyroyal

Pentachlorophenol

Pepcid

Pepino

Pepperoni

Peppers

Perch

Perfumes

ITEMS TO BE AVOIDED WITH PLD

PerioBrite toothpaste

Pesticides

Pheasant, commercial

Phenacetin

Phenols - nonylphenol / Phenosulfothiazine / Phenoxyethanol cosmetics

Phthalates plasticizers

Physalis peruviana (poha)

Phytates phytic acid

Phytoestrogens i.e. soy

Pickle juice / Pickled egg / Pickles

Pie: made with lard, sugar, wheat

Piloncillo

Piña colada

ITEMS TO BE AVOIDED WITH PLD

Pink meats: bacon, bologna, hot dog

Pink slime

Pioglitazone (wait)

Pita / Pita chips / Pizza wheat

Plastic all / Plastic wrap

Plum

PLX5568

Poha berry

Poke (raw fish)

Poke root

Polychlorinated biphenyls / Polycyclic aromatic hydrocarbons (PAHs) / Polyethylene

Pomegranate / juice caution

Poppadum

ITEMS TO BE AVOIDED WITH PLD

Poppyseed

Popsicles with sugar

Pork / Pork pie / Pork sausage / Portuguese sausage

Potato

Potato chips

Poultry commercial dipped in chlorine bath

Pregnancy

Premarin / Prempro

Prep lyte

Prepared packaged foods

Pretzels salted wheat

Prime rib

Priment dioica / Pimento

ITEMS TO BE AVOIDED WITH PLD

Processed American cheese / Processed foods
Produce dipped in chlorine bath
Progesterone
Progesterone & cream
Prosciutto
Provolone cheese
Prune / Prune butter / Prune juice
Pudding
PUFA Polyunsaturated fatty acids
Pumpkin pie whipped cream
Pumpkin seed/oil
Purelax
PureVia

ITEMS TO BE AVOIDED WITH PLD

Puri

PVC polyvinyl chloride

Quail / Quail eggs

Quarter pounder

Queen Anne's lace (wild carrot)

Raclette

Ractopamine

Ragu sauce

Ragwort

Rambutan

Ramen noodles

Rapadura

Ravioli

ITEMS TO BE AVOIDED WITH PLD

Raw egg whites / Raw eggs

Ready eat vegetables dipped in chlorine bath

Red clover tea/honey

Red food dyes

Red meat

Red pimento

Red velvet cake

Red white potato

Red yeast rice caution ↑ arsenic

Redbush

Reggiano cheese

Remifemin

Resveratrol

ITEMS TO BE AVOIDED WITH PLD

Revlon colorstay bronzer for the face

Rhatany

Rhubarb / Rice white caution ↑ arsenic

Rice ice cream (√ carrageenan) / Rice syrup / Rice wine

Rigatoni

Rindswurst

Roast beef pre-cooked

Rolls yeasted

Rolly toothpaste brush

Romano cheese

Root beer

Rosemary

Rum scotch gin methanol

ITEMS TO BE AVOIDED WITH PLD

Russet potato

S-adensylmethionine

Saccharin

Safflower oil

Sage

Saké

Salami

Salmon farmed esp. harmful

Salt limit

Salt pork

Saltines

Sambucol whole fruit

SAMe

ITEMS TO BE AVOIDED WITH PLD

Saran wrap

Sardines

Sarsaparilla

Sarsaparilla drinks

Sashimi

Sassafras / Sassafras drinks

Satureoides (Macela Achyrocline)

Sausage

Saw palmetto

Scallops

Scampi

Scar bio oil

Scent fragrance

ITEMS TO BE AVOIDED WITH PLD

Scrambled / eggs /egg white avitamin

Sea bass / Seaweed ↑ mercury

Seitan

Senna

Sesame seeds/Shampoo   with methylparabens

Shampoo with formaldehyde/with methylisothiazoline MIT

Shampoo with parabens/with phthalates / with sodium lauryl sulfate

Shark / Shell fish / Shrimp ↑ mercury

Shea butter endocrine disruptor

Siberian ginseng

Silver amalgam

Sirolimus

Skullcap

ITEMS TO BE AVOIDED WITH PLD

Sloppy Joe's

Smoothies with dairy sugar

Snakeroot

Soap powders

Soda pop

Sodium bicarbonate frequently

Sodium lauryl sulfate

Softlax

Solé

Solvents

Sorbitol

Sorrel dip in boiling water ↓ oxalates

Sour cream (√ carrageenan)

ITEMS TO BE AVOIDED WITH PLD

Soursop / Soy sauce

Soy / Soy bean oil / Soy flour / Soy lecithin/ Soy milk (√ carrageenan)

Spaghetti meat balls / meat sauce / Spaghetti sauce / Spaghetti wheat

SPAM

Spare ribs

Spices caution aflatoxin

Spiker water resistant styling glue

Spinach / Spinach apple juice / caution ↑oxalates

Spirits methanol

Spirulina

Splenda

Spray cleaners

Sprouts alfalfa / clover / soy

ITEMS TO BE AVOIDED WITH PLD

Squab commercial

Squid

St. John's Wort

Star anise

Starfruit

Statins (if possible)

Steak

Stephania tetrandra

Stevia

Stout malt liquor

Strawberry / Strawberry drinks

Stroganoff

Stuffing with wheat

ITEMS TO BE AVOIDED WITH PLD

Styrofoam containers

Sucanat / Sucralose / Sucrose / Sugar / Sugar cane

Sugar cane juice / Sugar cane crystals

Sugar cookies

Sunflower oil

Sunflower seeds

Sunscreen 4-Methylbenzylidene / Sunscreen benzophenone-3

Sushi / Sunett

Swedish meat balls

Sweet clover

Sweet One / Sweet'N Low

Swordfish ↑ mercury

Syzygium aromaticum (clove)

ITEMS TO BE AVOIDED WITH PLD

Syzygium malaccense (Mt. apple)

T'u-san-chi

Table sugar / Tagatose sugar

Tacos

Tagamet

Tagliatelle

Tahini

Tamales lard tomatoes

Tamari

Tamarind

Tania leaves

Tanqueray / Tequila

Tansy

ITEMS TO BE AVOIDED WITH PLD

Tarragon

Tea black / caffeine / decaffeinated / green / white

Tea tree oil

Teeth plastic fillings

Teflon

Tempé

Teriyaki sauce

Testosterone

Tilefish ↑ mercury

Tiramasu

TMAO Trimethylamine N-oxide

Tobacco

Tofu

ITEMS TO BE AVOIDED WITH PLD

Toll house cookies

Tom's toothpaste

Tomato / Tomato juice / Tomatoes canned BHT methanol

Tortellini

Tortillas wheat

Tree nuts caution aflatoxin

Trehalose (mycose) sugar

Tribulus Terrestris

Triclosan in drinking water

TriLyte

Triptolide (wait)

Trout ↑ mercury / Tuna ↑ mercury

Truvia / Turbinado sugar

ITEMS TO BE AVOIDED WITH PLD

Turkey commercial /Turkey bacon / Turkey sausage

Tylenol

Udon (Buckwheat + wheat)

Uva Ursi

V8

Valerian

Vanilla extract

Veal

Vegemite

Vegetable juice bottled/canned BPA/ canned methanol

Velveeta cheese

Vichyssoise

Vienna sausage

ITEMS TO BE AVOIDED WITH PLD

Vinegar

Vitamin K2 with soy

Vitex agnus-castus

Walnuts caution aflatoxin

Water crackers

Wax jambu

Weed killer

Wheat / Wheat germ / Wheatena

Whey

White chocolate

White flour, rice / White sugar beet sugar / White sugar cane sugar

White tea

Whiting/Wild boar/Wild carrot

ITEMS TO BE AVOIDED WITH PLD

Wild yam progesterone cream / Willow bark

Windex / Window cleaners

Wine /Withania somnifera

Wolfberry

Wonton

Wood ear fungus

Woodruff

Worcestershire sauce

Wormseed

Wormwood

Xagave

Xenoestrogens

Xylitol sugar / Xylitol spry toothpaste

ITEMS TO BE AVOIDED WITH PLD

Yeast / Yeasted baked goods / Yeasted breads
Yellow cheese
Yerba maté
Yerba maté
Yogurt made with dairy
Yucca
Zucchini if GMO

Avoid Herbs

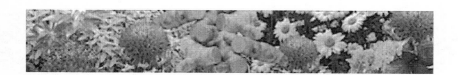

AVOID HERBS WITH PLD

Acacia fiber

Açai herb

Achyrocline

Aesculus hippocastanum

African autumn tea

African nectar tea

Agave cactus

Allspice

Aloe vera

Angelica dong quai

Annatto

Aristolochia

Ashwagandha

Aspergillus

Autumn crocus only if needed by prescription

Basil

Bearberry

Bilberry

Black cohosh

Black pepper caution aflatoxin

Black seed

Borage

Brahmi

Buchu

AVOID HERBS WITH PLD

Buckthorn

Bust enhancing herbs

Calendula

Callilepis laureola (Impila)

Cascara sagrada

Catchweed

Cats claw

Catsfoot

Cayenne pepper

Celandine

Celery leaf

Chaparral

Chaste-tree berry

Chervil

Chili caution aflatoxin

Chinese herbs

Chokeberry

Chrysanthemum

Cleavers

Clover

Cloves

Cohosh

Cola nut

Colchicine only if needed by prescription

Coleus

Coltsfoot

Comfrey ↓ liver functioning

Corydalis

AVOID HERBS WITH PLD

Country mallow

Dandelion greens

Devil's claw

Dill

Dong quai

Elderberry whole fruit

Ephedra sinica

Eugenol (oil of cloves)

Fennel

Fenugreek

Flaxseed

Fo ti

Forskolin

Galium aparine (cleavers)

Garcinia cambogia

Germander

Ginger ↑BP

Ginkgo biloba

Ginseng ↑BP

Goji

Goldenseal

Goosegrass

Gotu kola

Groundsel

Guarana

Harpagophytum

Hawthorne ↑BP

AVOID HERBS WITH PLD

Hops

Horse chestnut

Horseradish

Horsetail

Huckleberry

Impila root

Ivy

Jin Bu Huan

Juniper

Kava-kava

Keishi-bukuryo

Kola nut

Krameria triandra (rhatany root)

Kudzu

Kwao krua kao

Lavender

Lei gong teng (Wait)

Lemon verbena

Licorice ↑BP

Lobelia

Lupin

Ma Huang

Maca herb

Mace

Macela achyrocline satureoides

Magnolia officinalis

Mate

AVOID HERBS WITH PLD

Melaleuca

Mistletoe

Motherwort

Myristica fragrans

Nigella sativa

Noni

Nutmeg

Osha root

Paprika

Parsley ↑ oxalates ↓BP

Pau d'arco

Pennyroyal

Pimenta dioica

Pimento

Poke Root

Poppyseed

Queen Anne's lace (wild carrot)

Ragwort

Red clover

Redbush

Remifemin

Rhatany

Rooibos

Rosemary

Sage

Salt limit

Sarsaparilla

Sassafras

AVOID HERBS WITH PLD

Satureoides (Macela Achyrocline)

Saw palmetto

Senna

Siberian ginseng

Skullcap

Snakeroot

Sorrel

Spices caution aflatoxin

St. John's Wort

Star anise

Stephania tetrandra

Sunflower seed

Stevia

Stickyweed

Sweet clover

Syzygium aromaticum (clove)

T'u-san-chi

Tamarind

Tania leaves

Tansy

Tarragon

Tea plant

Tea tree oil

Thymoquinone

Tribulus Terrestris

Uva Ursi

Valerian

AVOID HERBS WITH PLD

Vanilla extract

Vitex agnus-castus

Wild carrot

Wild yam

Willow bark

Withania somnifera

Woodruff

Wormseed

Wormwood

Yerba mate

Yucca

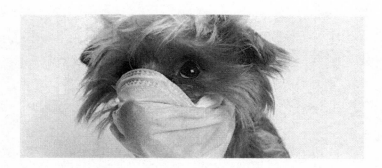

Chemicals to be Avoided

CHEMICALS TO BE AVOIDED

3-benzylidene-camphor

4-Methylbenzylidene-sunscreen

Acacia fiber

Acesulfame potassium

Acetaminophen

Acetylsalicylic acid

Acrylamide

ADA azobiscarbonaye diazenedicarboxamide

Advil

Aflatoxin

CHEMICALS TO BE AVOIDED

Agave

Aging (NMN)

Air fresheners phthalates

Alcohol

Alcohol aerosol

Alcohol methanol

Aldomet

Aleve

Algae

Alkylphenols

Aluminum

Amalgam silver teeth fillings

Amino acid L-arginine

Amino Acid L-canavanine

Amino acid L-carnitine

CHEMICALS TO BE AVOIDED

Amiodarone

Ammonia

Anabolic steroids

Anti-inflammatory medication

Antifreeze

Apple hard cider

Arabitol

Arganat natural clay toothpaste

Arginine

Arsenic

Artificial sweetener

Aspartame (Nutrasweet)

Aspirin

Assugrin

Atrazine (weedkiller)

CHEMICALS TO BE AVOIDED

Aveeno Baby Natural Mineral Block Face Stick

Azocarbonamide

Baking soda taken regularly

Bathroom sprays

BGH bovine growth hormone

BHA Butylated Hydroxyanisole

BHT Butylated hydroxytoluene

Bio-oil

Birth control pills

Bisacodyl

Bisphenol A plastic

Bleach

Bleach cleanser

Blue-green algae

Bontanique toothpaste

CHEMICALS TO BE AVOIDED

Bottled juices methanol

Bovine growth hormone BGH

BPA bisphenol A plastic

Bragg's liquid aminos

Brake fluid

Bud-nip

Butylated hydroxyanisole/BHA

Cadium

Caffeine

cAMP

Canavanine

Canned goods ↑ methanol

Carbamazepine

Carbon tetrachloride

Carnitine

CHEMICALS TO BE AVOIDED

Carrageenan

Cascara sagrada

Casein

Chemicals ↑ cough

Chitosan

Chlorella

Chloride

Chlorine comet

Chlorpropham

Chondroitin

Cigarettes cigars chewing tobacco

Cimetidine

Cleanser with bleach

ClearLax

Clenz-Lyte

CHEMICALS TO BE AVOIDED

Co-Lav

Cod liver oil

Colase®

Colax

Colgate toothpaste

Colovage

CoLyte

Comet cleanser

Constipation

Coral calcium

Coral white toothpaste

Cordarone (Amiodarone)

Cordyceps (fungi)

Cosmetics phenooxyethanol

Cosmetics with cod liver oil

CHEMICALS TO BE AVOIDED

Cottonseed oil

Cranberry pills

Cream of tartar

Creatine supplements

Crest toothpaste

Crisco

Cyclamate

Daptacel vaccine (Phenoxyethanol)

DCA Dichloroacetate in tap water

DDD Dichlorodiphenyldichloroethane

DDE insecticide residue

DDT insecticide

DEHP (PVC plasticizer)

Detergents

Dichloroacetate DCA

CHEMICALS TO BE AVOIDED

Dichlorodiphenyldichloroethane

Deldrin insecticide

Diethyl phthalate

Diethylstilbestrol estrogen

Diflucan

Doxidan

DPA Diphenylamine

DPT Diphenylthiazole

Dry cleaned chemical/clothing

Dryer sheets

Dulcolax

E-Z-Em Fortrans

Ecstasy

Endocrine disruptors

Endosulfan (insecticide)

CHEMICALS TO BE AVOIDED

Ephedra

Equal

Erythritol

Erythrosine FD&C Red #3

Estrace

Estrogen

Estrogen BCP/pill/patch

Estrogen disruptors

Estrogenic shampoos

Ethanol

Ethylene glycol

Excedrin

Fabric softener

Face cream

Famotidine

CHEMICALS TO BE AVOIDED

Fish cod liver oil

Fish oil

Flagyl

Flaxseed oil capsules

Fluconazole

Fluoride

Foods heated in plastic

Formaldehyde

Forskolin

Fragrance

Fragrance: BHT endocrine disruptor

Fragrance: Diethyl phthalate mimics hormones

Fragrance: Limonene can create formaldehyde

Fragrance: Octinoxate endocrine disruptor

Fragrance: Oxybenzone endocrine disruptor

CHEMICALS TO BE AVOIDED

Galactitol

Garcinia cambodia

GaviLax

Gavilyte

Gelatin

Genistein (soy)

Gentamycin

Glucosamine

Glycolax

Glycols polyethylene → polyester

GlycoPrep

GMO

GMO seed

Go-Evac

GoLYTELY®

CHEMICALS TO BE AVOIDED

Hair chemicals dye

Hair gel

HalfLytely

Heating food in microwave

Heptachlor (instecticide)

Herbicides

High fructose corn syrup HFCS

Homocysteine

Hormones HRT

HRT hormones replacement estrogen

Hydrogenated starch hydrolysate

Hydrolyzed wheat protein

Ibuprofen

Imitrex

Inflammation

CHEMICALS TO BE AVOIDED

Isomalt

Jason Oral comfort toothpaste

Jason PowerSmile toothpaste

Juice bottled methanol / Juice canned BPA

Just like sugar

Ketoconazole

Kiss my face toothpaste

Kombucha

L-arginine

L-canavanine

L-carnitine

L'oreal HiP High Intensity Pigments

Lactitol

Lard

Laundry powder (inhaling)

CHEMICALS TO BE AVOIDED

Lax-a-Day

Laxatives

LaxLyte

Lead

Lecithin (soy)

Lectin

Lesys (Maltitol, MaltiSweet, SweetPearl)

Limonene→ formaldehyde

Lindane (insecticide)

Linseed

Lithium

Lollipops

Lupin

Lysergic Acid LSD

LytePrep

CHEMICALS TO BE AVOIDED

Macrogol

Maltisweet (Maltitol Lesys SweetPearl)

Maltitiol

Mannitol

Margarine

Mederma

Menaquinone w/soy

Mercury

Metalloestrogens

Methanol

Methanol alcoholic drinks

Methionine

Methoxychlor (insecticide)

Methyldopa

Methylisothiazoline

CHEMICALS TO BE AVOIDED

Methylparabens

Microwaved food

Migraine

MiraLAX

MIT Methylisothiazolinone

Mixed alcoholic methanol

MK-7 w/soy

Monster drink

Motrin

Movicol

MoviPrep

MSG (monosodium glutamate)

MSM (methylsulfonylmethane)

Multiple vitamins

Muscovado sugar

CHEMICALS TO BE AVOIDED

Mycose

N-nitrosomorpholine NNM

Nail chemicals polish removers

Naltrexone

Naproxen

Nattōkinase

Nattō

Natural dentist toothpaste

Natural tea tree oil toothpaste

Neatsfoot oil

Nectresse

Neem toothpaste

Neotame

Neutrogena body oil

Neutrogena liquid facial cleanser fragrance free

CHEMICALS TO BE AVOIDED

Nitrites
Nitrosamine
Nizoral
NNM (N-nitrosomorpholine)
Non-dairy creamer
Non-stick teflon
Nonylphenol derivatives
Norbu
NSAIDs
NuLYTELY
NutraSweet (aspartame)
Nutribiotic toothpaste
Nutritional yeast
OCL (laxative)
Octinoxate

CHEMICALS TO BE AVOIDED

Olay Daily Facials Deep Cleansing Cloths

Organic chlorines pesticides

Ospemifene

Osphena®

Oven cleaners

Oxybenzone

PAHs Polycyclic aromatic hydrocarbons

Palm oil

Parabens

Paracetamol

Peg Lyte

Pentachlorophenol

Pepcid

Perfumes

PerioBrite toothpaste

CHEMICALS TO BE AVOIDED

Pesticides

Phenacetin

Phenols - nonylphenol

Phenosulfothiazine

Phenoxyethanol cosmetics

Phthalates plasticizers

Phytates phytic acid

Phytoestrogens i.e. soy

Pink slime

Pioglitazone (wait)

Plastic

Plastic wrap

Plexxicon

PLX5568

Polychlorinated biphenyls

CHEMICALS TO BE AVOIDED

Polycyclic aromatic hydrocarbons PAHs

Polyester

Polyethylene glycol

Pregnancy

Premarin

Prempro

Prep lyte

Progesterone

PUFA Polyunsaturated fatty acids

Purelax

PureVia

PVC Polyvinyl chloride

Ractopamine

Red food dye

Red yeast rice caution ↑ arsenic

CHEMICALS TO BE AVOIDED

Remifemin
Resveratrol
Reversin
Revlon ColorStay Bronzer for the Face
Rice wine caution ↑ arsenic
Rolly toothpaste brush
Roscovitine
Roundup®
Rum scotch gin methanol
S-adensylmethionine
Saccharin
Saké
SAMe
Saran wrap
Scar oil

CHEMICALS TO BE AVOIDED

Scent fragrance

Seliciclib

Shampoo with formaldehyde

Shampoo with methylisothiazoline MIT

Shampoo with methylparabens

Shampoo with parabens

Shampoo with phthalates

Shampoo with sodium lauryl sulfate

Silver amalgam

Sirolimus

Soap powders

Sodium bicarbonate frequently

Sodium lauryl sulfate

Softlax

Solvents

CHEMICALS TO BE AVOIDED

Sorbitol

Soy lecithin

Soy sauce

Spiker water resistant styling glue

Spirits

Spirulina

Splenda

Spray cleaners

Statins if possible

Stevia

Stout malt liquor

Styrofoam containers

Sucanat

Sucralose

Sucrose

CHEMICALS TO BE AVOIDED

Sugar cane crystals

Sugar twin

Sunett

Sunflower oil

Sunscreen 4-Methylbenzylidene

Sunscreen benzophenone-3

Sweet One

Sweet'N Low

SweetPearl (maltitol)

Table sugar

Tagamet

Tagatose sugar

Tamari

Tanqueray

Teeth plastic fillings

CHEMICALS TO BE AVOIDED

Teflon
Tempeh
Tequila
Teriyaki sauce
Testosterone
Thymoquinone
TMAO Trimethylamine N-oxide
Tobacco
Tom's toothpaste
Trehalose sugar
Triclosan in water supply
TriLyte
Triptolide (wait)
Truvia
Turbinado sugar

CHEMICALS TO BE AVOIDED

Tylenol

Vegemite

Vinegar

Vitamin K2 w/soy

Weedkiller

Whey

Wild yam progesterone cream

Windex

Window cleaners

Wine

Worcestershire sauce

Xagave

Xanthan gum

Xenoestrogens

Xylitol

CHEMICALS TO BE AVOIDED

Xylitol Spry toothpaste

Yeast

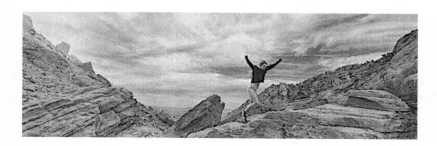

Everyone to Avoid

EVERYONE TO AVOID

Aluminum
Artificial sweeteners
Candy
Crisco
French fries
Lard
Margarine
Peanuts
Potato chips
Processed foods

EVERYONE TO AVOID

White flour and sugar

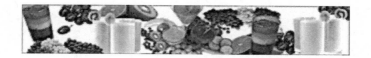

Drinks to Avoid

DRINKS AVOID

Açai smoothie

African autumn tea

African nectar tea

Alcohol

Ale

Apple hard cider with sugar

Beer

Black tea

Bottled juice

Caffeinated drinks

Cane juice

Canned drinks

Canned juice esp ↑ methanol

Cappuccino

Carbonated soda

Celery juice

Chaga mushroom tea

Chaparral tea

Chocolate drinks milk

Clam juice

DRINKS AVOID

Coca cola

Cocktails

Cocoa caution aflatoxin

Coffee

Cola drinks

Cream

Dairy caution aflatoxin

Decaf coffee

Decaf colas

Decaf drinks

Decaf tea

Dr. Pepper

Egg raw

Egg white raw

Eggnog

Energy drink

Ensure

Espresso

Ethanol

Ginger ale

Grain beverage bambu

DRINKS AVOID

Grain beverage faux joe

Grain beverage postum

Grain beverage soyfee

Grain beverage yannoh

Grapefruit juice caution

Green leaf tea

Hard cider

Harmful herb tea African autumn

Harmful herb tea African nectar

Harmful herb tea apple chamomile

Harmful herb tea Bengal spice

Harmful herb tea black cherry berry

Harmful herb tea caffeine free

Harmful herb tea chaparral

Harmful herb tea chocolate mint truffle

Harmful herb tea chrysanthemum

Harmful herb tea cinnamon apple spice

Harmful herb tea country peach

Harmful herb tea cranberry apple zinger

Harmful herb tea essiac

Harmful herb tea fast lane black

DRINKS AVOID

Harmful herb tea fennel seed tea

Harmful herb tea guarana

Harmful herb tea honeybush

Harmful herb tea honeyVanillaChamomile

Harmful herb tea jammin lemon ginger

Harmful herb tea lemon herbal love lemon

Harmful herb tea lemon verbena

Harmful herb tea lemon zinger

Harmful herb tea licorice root

Harmful herb tea maca

Harmful herb tea mama bear's cold care

Harmful herb tea mandarin orange

Harmful herb tea metabo balance

Harmful herb tea morning thunder

Harmful herb tea raspberry zinger

Harmful herb tea red clover

Harmful herb tea red tea

Harmful herb tea red zinger

Harmful herb tea redbush

Harmful herb tea roastaroma

Harmful herb tea rooibos

DRINKS AVOID

Harmful herb tea rooibos chai

Harmful herb tea sarsaparilla

Harmful herb tea sassafras

Harmful herb tea sleepytime

Harmful herb tea sleepytime grape

Harmful herb tea sleepytime peach

Harmful herb tea sleepytime vanilla

Harmful herb tea tangerine zinger

Harmful herb tea tension tamer

Harmful herb tea true blueberry

Harmful herb tea wild berry zinger

Harmful herb tea yerba mate

Harmful tea black

Harmful tea caffeine

Harmful tea Chinese gunpowder tea

Harmful tea decaffeinated

Harmful tea Earl Gray tea

Harmful tea green tea

Harmful white tea

Hot chocolate

Hot toddy

DRINKS AVOID

Juice bottled/canned BPA

Lassi

Latté

Licorice drinks

Mai tai

Malt liquors

Mangosteen bottled juice

Methanol

Methanol alcoholic drinks

Mexican hot chocolate

Milk cow, goat, animal

Milk shakes animal milk

Mixed alcohol

Mixed alcoholic drinks methanol

Monster energy drink

Noni juice

Pickle juice

Piña colada

Pomegranate juice

Prune juice

Raw egg whites

DRINKS AVOID

Raw eggs

Rice wine caution ↑ arsenic

Root beer

Rum scotch gin methanol

Saké

Sarsaparilla drinks

Sassafras drinks

Smoothies with dairy sugar

Spinach apple juice

Soda pop

Soy milk

Spirits

Stout malt liquor

Strawberry drinks

Sugar cane juice

Tanqueray

Tea black

Tea caffeine

Tea decaffeinated

Tea white

Tequila

DRINKS AVOID

Tomato juice

V8

Veg juice bottle/canned BPA

Wine

Yogurt drinks with sugar and dairy

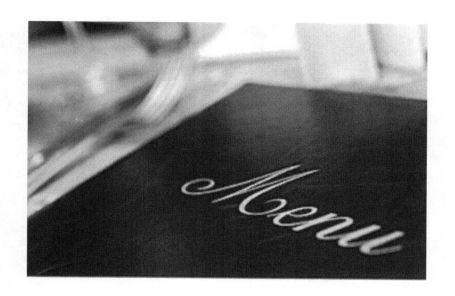

MENUS

Recipe inspirations
PKDrecipes.com

Upon Arising Menu

One teaspoon of solé in a glass of water.

After eating raw fruit or drinking citrus, please allow 20 minutes before taking something else.

Freshly squeezed lemon juice, add just enough water to make $\frac{1}{4}$ cup; please allow 20 minutes before taking something else.

Freshly squeezed orange juice; please allow 20 minutes before taking something else.

Grapefruit juice freshly squeezed (caution interferes with many medications); please allow 20 minutes before taking something else.

Throughout the day, if permitted, drink water equal to twice your output (or ~4Liters) thus turning off vasopressin, a hormone that stimulates cyst growth.

Breakfast Menu

After eating raw fruit or drinking citrus, please allow 20 minutes before taking something else.

Breakfast Menu

Fruit: Raw fresh fruit in season & locally grown: banana, figs, kiwi, kumquats, pear, grapefruit, apple, clementine or if in the tropics: mango, papaya, jack fruit (the biggest and one of the sweetest fruits in the world and it hangs ripening from a majestic tree), pomelo, cherimoya. During berry season a bowl filled with ripe red raspberries, black raspberries and blackberries from the wild might be a start for the day.

Strawberries are too acid forming joining fruits to be avoided: starfruit, rhubarb, strawberry, plum, prunes, rambutan, poha berry, lychee, longan, ackee.

Fruit: Freshly sliced grapefruit (caution grapefruit interferes with certain medications).

Fruit: Bananas and apples or stewed fruit.

Fruit: Freshly squeezed orange juice

Cereal: Corn meal with chopped dates. Soak grains overnight.

Cereal: Hot cereal made from spelt, rye, kamut, grits, corn meal, steel cut oats or oatmeal with almond, coconut, hempseed, barley, or oat milk.

Breakfast Menu

Hot cereal: Prepare ½ cup of spelt kernels that have been soaked overnight to diminish phytic acid. Whole spelt kernels have a taste similar to a bowl of ground nuts. Grind the kernels in a food processor. The following morning heat and top with banana, dates, pears, or cinnamon apples.

Toasted non-yeasted English Muffin spelt, rye, kamut, brown rice~caution ↑ arsenic, corn with an all fruit spread or almond butter or both.

Toasted non-yeasted non-wheat bread spelt, rye, kamut, brown rice~caution ↑ arsenic, corn with an all fruit spread or almond butter or both.

Toasted non-yeasted non-wheat bagel: spelt, rye, kamut, brown rice~caution ↑ arsenic, corn.

Warmed non-yeasted pita: spelt, rye, kamut, corn stuffed with chopped cilantro, garlic, and avocado.

Warmed non-yeasted Baps: spelt, rye, kamut, corn stuffed with chopped cilantro, garlic, and avocado.

Warmed non-yeasted pita: spelt, rye, kamut, corn stuffed with chopped cilantro garlic, and avocado.

Toasted non-yeasted non-wheat bread spelt, rye, kamut, brown rice~caution ↑ arsenic, corn with sautéed mushrooms, almond butter, cashew butter, bean spread, or avocado are a few alternative spreads.

Essene bread spread with almond butter.

Breakfast Menu

Warmed corn tortillas; homemade spelt chapattis or another non-yeasted flat breads such as parathas, crackers, and spelt dosas. These taste so much better when freshly prepared by yourself without yeast.

Waffle, crêpes, pancakes made from spelt, rye, kamut, corn grains and without eggs or yeast.

Non-yeasted breads made with spelt, rye, kamut, corn, brown rice~caution ↑ arsenic: the dough is a flour and water mixture. This rises for 7 hours before baked. Unlike yeasted breads which rise quickly; non-yeasted breads release their digestive enzymes in the lactic acid ferment. This lactic acid can be blown off by several deep breaths throughout the day. Other acids produced by the body increase the workload upon cystic kidneys, this in turn affects the liver. After eating non-yeasted spelt bread many have noticed that they never come away with a bloated feeling. It is similar when soaking nuts, beans, legumes and seeds to lessen their phytic acid content. With large ever expanding cystic organs, it is very useful to minimize bloating. Many with liver cysts take H2 blockers. In theory this slows down secretin and prevents liver cysts from expanding.

Liquids: enjoy following solid food. Eat a raw slice of alkaline fruit twenty minutes before a meal. After eating raw fruit or drinking citrus, please allow 20 minutes before taking something else.

Breakfast Menu

Herb Tea Chamomile, chamomile citrus, hibiscus, lemon grass, lemon thyme, lemon water, linden flower, milk thistle, rose hips, saffron tea, silymarin, sugar cookie sleigh ride, thyme, tilleul, or veronica tea.

Roasted grain beverage: barley brew, barley cup, cafix, caro, carob powder, inka, java herb uncoffee, kara kara, organic instant grain, prewetts chicory, roma, spelt kaffee, or teeccino.

Water: Lemon water, mineral water, spring water or water that has been left out for 24 hours to dissipate any residual chlorine.

Lunch Menu

Soup: Lentil or bean soup with brown rice. Caution rice may contain arsenic.

Soup: Coconut milk mixed with vegetables and brown rice. Caution rice may contain arsenic.

Soup sides: spelt bread, spelt crackers, corn tortillas, brown rice crackers. Caution rice products may contain arsenic.

Lunch Menu

Salad: romaine lettuce, sliced radish, diced carrot, purple onion, mushrooms, jicama, turnip (quick dip leafy greens in hot water or lemon to diminish any residual oxalates).

Sandwich: Almond vegetable paté on non-yeasted spelt, kamut, or as hor d'oeuvres or corn bread. This spread can be also be placed on a round sliced cucumber or zucchini.

Sandwich: Vegetable burger made without soy or wheat on non-yeasted spelt, kamut, or a corn bread bun.

Sandwich: Almond butter and fruit spread or sliced banana.

Sandwich: Avocado radish sprout sandwich or warmed corn tortilla with avocado, onion, garlic, radish sprouts.

Sandwich: Pita with diced steamed vegetables (spelt, kamut, or corn pita).

Sandwich: Walnut vegetable paté lettuce, purple onion, cucumber.

Vegetables: Moroccan vegetable stew with beans that have been soaked for 3 days.

Vegetables: Vegetables wrapped in a romaine lettuce leaf.

Vegetables: Buddha's delight.

Liquids~enjoy liquids following eating solid food.

Lunch Menu

Herb Tea Chamomile, chamomile citrus, chocolate hibiscus, lemon grass, lemon thyme, lemon water, linden flower, milk thistle, rose hips, saffron tea, silymarin, sugar cookie sleigh ride, thyme, tilleul, or veronica tea.

Roasted grain beverage: barley brew, barley cup, cafix, caro, carob powder, inka, java herb uncoffee, kara kara, organic instant grain, prewetts chicory, roma, spelt kaffee or teeccino.

Water: Lemon water, mineral water, spring water or water that has been left out for 24 hours to dissipate any residual chlorine.

Dinner Menu

Raw spring roll with cubed carrots, onions, peas, radish, mint.

Pasta: spelt pasta fettuccine with roasted squash, chard, kale, almonds, garlic, lemon or spring onions.

Pie: Vegetable pie

Pie: Wild mushroom shepherd's pie made with root vegetables

Dinner Menu

Pizza spelt crust without yeast with mushrooms, onion, garlic, or parsley.

Polenta crispy with roasted vegetables

Vegetables: Roasted root vegetables: rutabagas, carrots, sweet potatoes, turnips, beets, and some above ground crops such as artichokes, carrots, or squash.

Vegetables: Steamed array of vegetables: corn, squash, onion, garlic, celeriac, pumpkin, sunchokes, artichokes.

Vegetables with brown rice~caution ↑ arsenic, squash risotto

Vegetables: Vegetables with spelt pasta. To diminish symptoms continue to avoid the nightshade plants of tomatoes, bell peppers, eggplant, potatoes.

Vegetables: All vegetable Terrine or Paté

Vegetables: All vegetable tagine chickpeas, saffron, cilantro over quinoa

Vegetables: Corn cakes with walnut sauce, braised oxblood carrots with spelt pasta.

Vegetables: Mushroom tart with leeks.

Vegetables: Curries cauliflower and peas with brown rice. Caution rice may contain arsenic.

Vegetables: Moroccan vegetable curry.

Dinner Menu

Vegetables: Slow roasted Okinawan sweet potatoes; braised carrots; steamed corn; sautéed leafy greens with currants, pine nuts, garlic, and lemon.

Vegetables: Brown rice~caution ↑ arsenic, and beans

Vegetables: Pot-au-feu made with all vegetables.

Liquids: Enjoy liquids after solid food: a cup of herb tea, nettle extract in warm water; thyme tea; veronica tea; grain beverage or water.

Late Night Snack

Water: Place water by the bed with a lemon slice if desired.

Juice: Grape juice (all juice) with 2 ounces of mineral water.

Juice: Cranberry (all juice) with 2 ounces of mineral water. If urine is too alkaline in the evening, cranberry juice will make it slightly more acidic.

Herb Tea Chamomile tea with tupelo honey if desired.

Liquids~enjoy liquids following eating solid food.

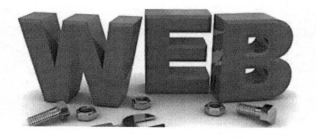

HELPFUL WEBSITES

Helpful Web Sites	
KIDNEY	Polycystic-KidneyDisease.com/index2.html
LIVER	www.PolycysticLiverDisease.com/index2.html
RECIPE INSPIRATIONS	www.PKDrecipes.com
PKD / PLD DETAILS	www.pkdiet.com/index2.php
ALKALINE DIET	http://www.AlkalineDiet.com

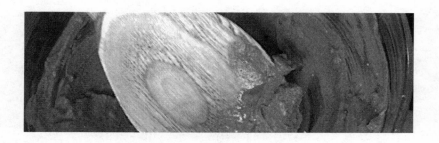

DERMATOLOGY SYMPTOMS

Sometimes we get itchy skin, thinning hair, whitened nails, cramping legs. Many personal care products aggravate polycystic liver symptoms or increase cyst growth. EWG http://www.ewg.org/skindeep/ has a database rating of many personal products.

To diminish itching try using bentonite clay paste in lieu of soap. While in the shower, apply olive oil on the skin.

Then under running water, rub on bentonite clay paste (recipe follows).

Wrap a sliced lemon in cheese cloth. Gently rub the cut surface of the wrapped lemon over the skin. Apply additional olive oil; rinse with water.

Sprinkle baking soda on wet skin to help remove any residual oil; a final rinse with copious amounts of water; then pat dry. These methods help ease itching and dry skin.

Bentonite clay paste

1 cup of clay

1 cup of olive oil (add sufficient oil to make a paste)
1 teaspoon of tupelo honey

Some have tried eliminating shampoo and using a clay hair masque.

Rhassoul (Ghassoul) Moroccan clay hair masque

Black rubber bowl used to mix plaster (3 cup size)

2 Tablespoons of red Moroccan clay

1-2 drops of burdock oil (Klettenwurzel Haar-Oil)

Wire whisk

Warm water

CAUTION olive oil can make shower surfaces very slippery.

Mix together the clay and oil to form a paste. Apply on damp hair. Leave on for about an hour. Then rinse. A few more suggestions are available.

http://www.polycystic-kidneydisease.com/html/pkd_dermatology.html

Some other things a few PLD'rs have found helpful: clay baths, saunas, artichokes, cabbage, DIMs (broccoli sprouts), milk thistle, saffron, sunchokes, and turmeric all increase the metabolism of estrogen.

Clay baths allow for utilization of the entire skin surface to help diminish liver toxins. Saunas allow the use of the body's surface as an organ to decrease toxins.

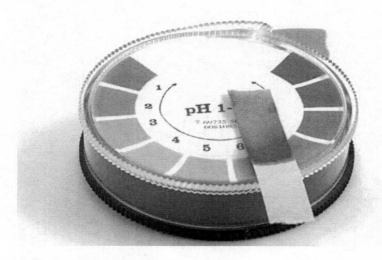

ALKALINE TRIAL

The time may be ideal for an Alkaline PLD Clinical Trial. 1998 research by the Tanners showed *Citrate Therapy Improved PKD Renal Function* http://www.pkdiet.com/pdf/kcitanner/kcit1998.pdf

In the year 2000, research showed that

Citrate Therapy or alkalinity improved PKD.

http://www.pkdiet.com/pdf/kcitanner/kcit2000.pdf

2010 - 2014   Alkaline Clinical Trials

http://www.polycysticliverdisease.com/pdf/AlkalineTrial.pdf

2010 Clinical Trial sodium citrate-alkalinity improves GFR

https://www.ncbi.nlm.nih.gov/pubmed/20072112

2010 Clinical Trial completed using potassium citrate in renal transplant patients

https://clinicaltrials.gov/ct2/show/NCT00913796

2010 Basic approach to chronic kidney disease

https://www.ncbi.nlm.nih.gov/pubmed/20224583

2010 Alkaline Diet reduces urinary oxalate excretion, prominent in PKD

https://www.ncbi.nlm.nih.gov/pubmed/20736987

2012 Potassium citrate helps manage uric acid

https://www.ncbi.nlm.nih.gov/pubmed/21858663

2010 Clinical Trial potassium citrate boosts bone density in the elderly

http://www.polycystic-kidneydisease.com/pdf/BoneDensity.pdf

2010 Veggie diet best for kidney patients

http://www.medpagetoday.com/Nephrology/GeneralNephrology/24060

2010 Clinical Trial: acid retention leads to progressive GFR decline, remedied by alkaline diet

http://www.medpagetoday.com/Nephrology/
GeneralNephrology/24060

2013 Clinical Trial: plant based protects against renal toxicity and loss of DNA integrity

http://www.pkdiet.com/pdf/AlkalineTrial/
PlantBasedDiet.pdf

2014 Plant Based MultiCenter Study Reduces Depression Anxiety & Improves Quality of Life

https://www.ncbi.nlm.nih.gov/pubmed/24524383

2014 Dietary Patterns Risk of Death Progression ESRD in Individuals with CKD: A Cohort

https://www.ncbi.nlm.nih.gov/pubmed/24679894

2014 Plant Based Diet Lowers Risk of Renal Cell Carcinoma in Large US Cohort Study

http://www.pkdiet.com/pdf/AlkalineTrial/
PlantFoodsRCC.pdf

2016 PKD Diet Low Osmolar Diet, The Water Diet

https://clinicaltrials.gov/ct2/show/NCT02225860?
term=polycystic+kidney&rank=40

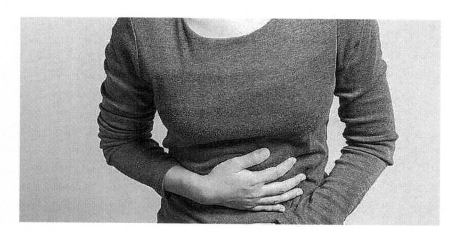

PLD PAIN

The most common question is what to do about PLD pain. This is the main thing that brings us to the doctor. We cannot use any over the counter pain relief.

Get to a PLD center so the doctors can help with pain relief. There are a few non-medication suggestion used by others with PLD.

http://www.pkdiet.com/pdf/lists/pain.pdf

Some clinical trials are underway to help with PLD pain. Do not let anyone talk you into that your PLD pain is not real. It is very real. Find someone who will give you help.

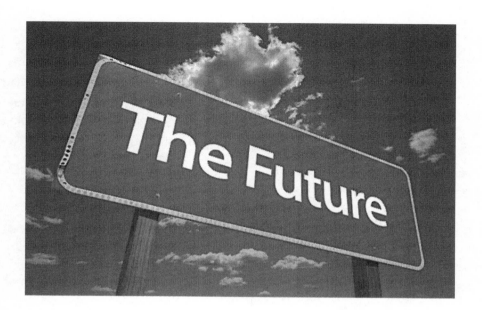

THE FUTURE

There are several clinical trials underway for PLD, mostly involving a drug like octreotide. Without a trial, the cost for a month is about $7000. Little polymers keep the drug within the body system for about 28 days. This is an injectable and this drug works as long as the injection lasts. We are hopeful and optimistic that in the foreseeable future a PLD Diet will become as commonplace as an adjunctive medical therapy for PLD; its utilization will become as clear-cut as incorporating a diabetic diet in the treatment of diabetes.

Clinging to the prospect that conceivably what may lie ahead for us is a home unit with the ability for testing of our electrolytes and alkalinity (similar to existing home blood sugar kits). We can imagine that the existence of such a machine could be coupled with the PLD Diet, bringing about true alkalinity and health for many with cystic organ disease.

No one is sure why or if alkalinity works for PLD. Our personal experience is that it is indeed helpful. A determination can be made through a clinical trial. Together, let us begin PLD alkaline trials. Let us dream and hope for a bright PLD future.

Made in the USA
San Bernardino, CA
13 October 2017